Red-Hot Sex
the Kama Sutra Way

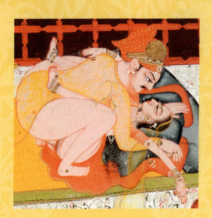

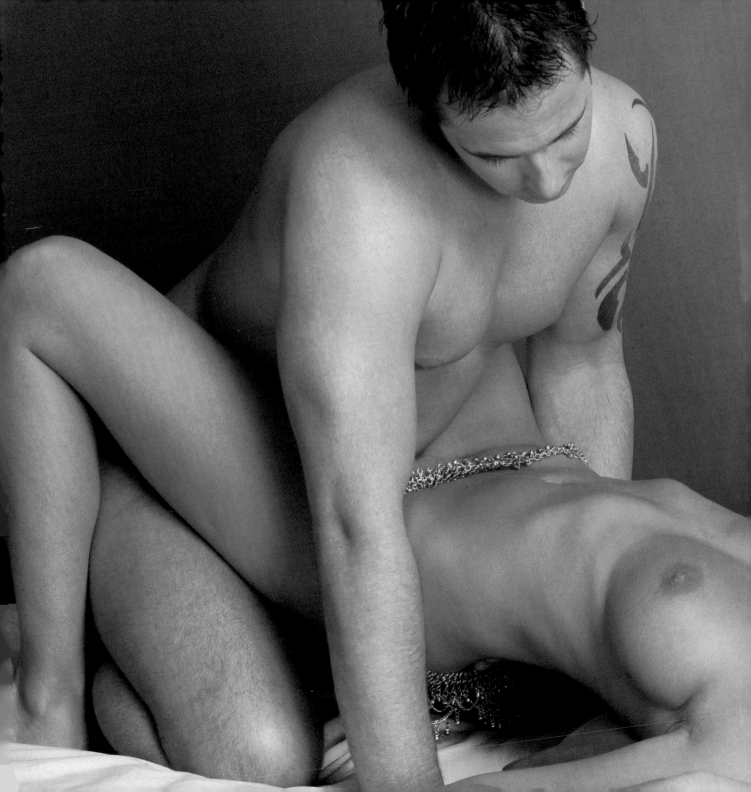

Red-Hot Sex the Kama Sutra Way

RICHARD EMERSON 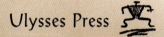 Ulysses Press

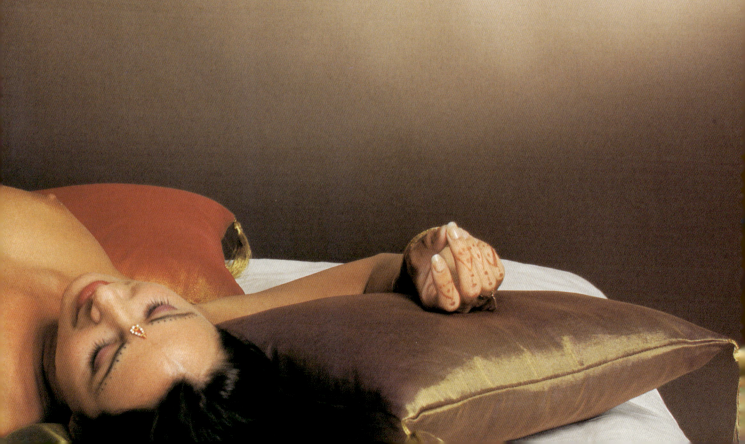

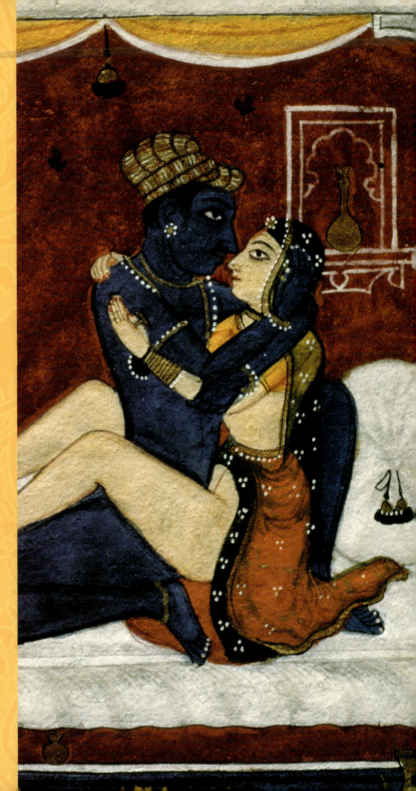

Text, design and illustration copyright © 2004 Carlton Books Limited. All rights reserved. No part of this publication may be reproduced, stored in a retrieval system, or transmitted in any form or by any means, electronic, mechanical, photocopying, recording or otherwise, without the prior permission of the copyright owner.

Published in the United States by
Ulysses Press
P.O. Box 3440
Berkeley, CA 94703
www.ulyssespress.com

ISBN 1-56975-463-2
Library of Congress Control Number 2004111117

First published as *The New Kama Sutra* in Great Britain in 2004 by Carlton Books Ltd.

Executive Editor: Lisa Dyer
Design: DW Design
Copy Editor: Jane Donovan
Picture Research: Sarah Edwards
Production Controller: Caroline Alberti

Printed and bound in Portugal

10 9 8 7 6 5 4 3 2

Distributed in the United States by Publishers Group West and in Canada by Raincoast Books

INTRODUCTION	6
THE TEACHINGS OF THE KAMA SUTRA	8
ATTRACTING A PARTNER	30
THE SEXUAL ENCOUNTER	50
SEXUAL POSITIONS	76
SEXUAL MAGIC	96
APPENDIX: SAFETY ISSUES AND SEXUAL PROBLEMS	114
INDEX	126
ACKNOWLEDGEMENTS	128

The book that became the guide to Tantric love and sex was written between 100 and 3300 AD by the Hindu philosopher Vatsyayana. The Kama Sutra exhorted followers to master their sexual impulses through becoming an expert in the arts of love. By conquering your sexuality, rather than letting its hormonal rush dominate your behaviour, you could win material, spiritual and amorous successes. Many of Vatsyayana's original recommendations are relevant in today's society, particularly the idea that the physical universe is matched by an invisible one of power and energy.

In the original Kama Sutra, men were encouraged to honour, cherish and love their partners; although this might sometimes appear to be sexist, the fact is that women were cherished and valued. The modern interpretation sees the sex act as a meeting of equals willing to share the life force that can flow between the two parties. For the man to succeed at love, he has to be adept at all aspects of making love, and that goes beyond the physical. He has to fully appreciate the beauty of what is around him, which includes being familiar with the disciplines of music and art. This approach to life and education is intended to give him a rounded character and make him interesting to a woman.

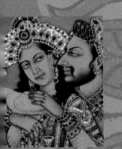

INTRODUCTION

The original text of the Kama Sutra speaks of the sixty-four arts. In just the same way that men and women today are expected to know how to text each other or communicate via e-mail, so men were expected to be competent in a wide range of activities to charm others while they passed the time of day. They were skilled in writing and drawing, painting, making stained glass, sewing, reading, composing tunes and songs, reciting poetry and etiquette. They were also adept at carpentry, gambling and martial arts, much as some men are today.

To have satisfying sex in modern society, we can learn from the edicts laid out thousands of years ago. A couple can begin their journey by awakening all the senses – touch, taste, scent, sound and sight. Both the man and the woman can take pleasure in the beauty around them: the food and drink they have prepared and laid out in an attractive way, the comfortable surroundings they have arranged, the music playing, the conversation.

These attentive actions are each an important part of the build-up to great sex. They create a harmony and a connection between the individuals, bringing the couple closer together. Sex is not the most important aspect of the relationship, but an integral part of the whole. The lesson that the ancient rites can teach us is to concentrate on each other, taking the time and space to be comfortable with and to please each other. It is as if you can explore the freshness of your relationship all over again by exploring new ideas and the physical body.

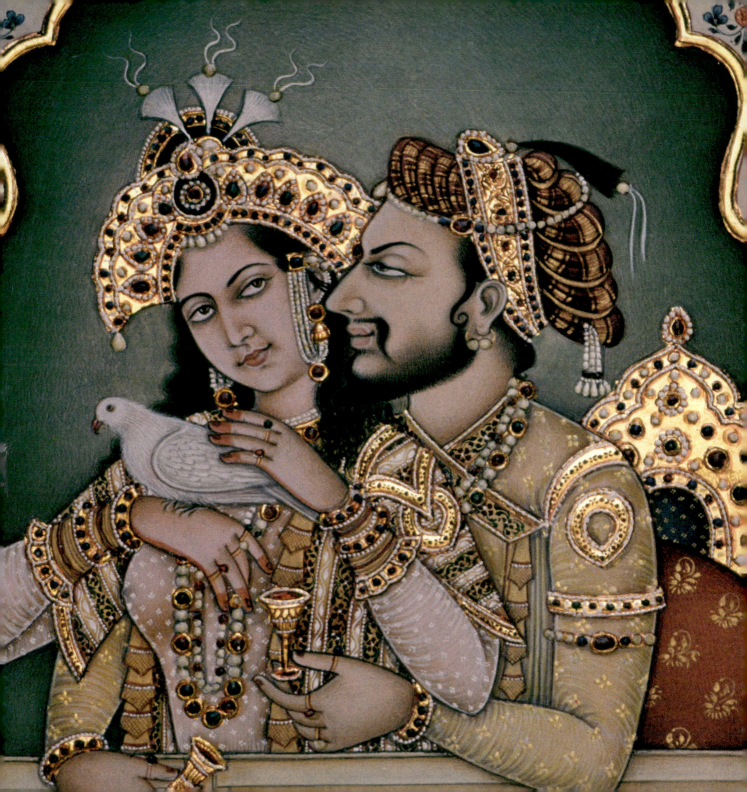

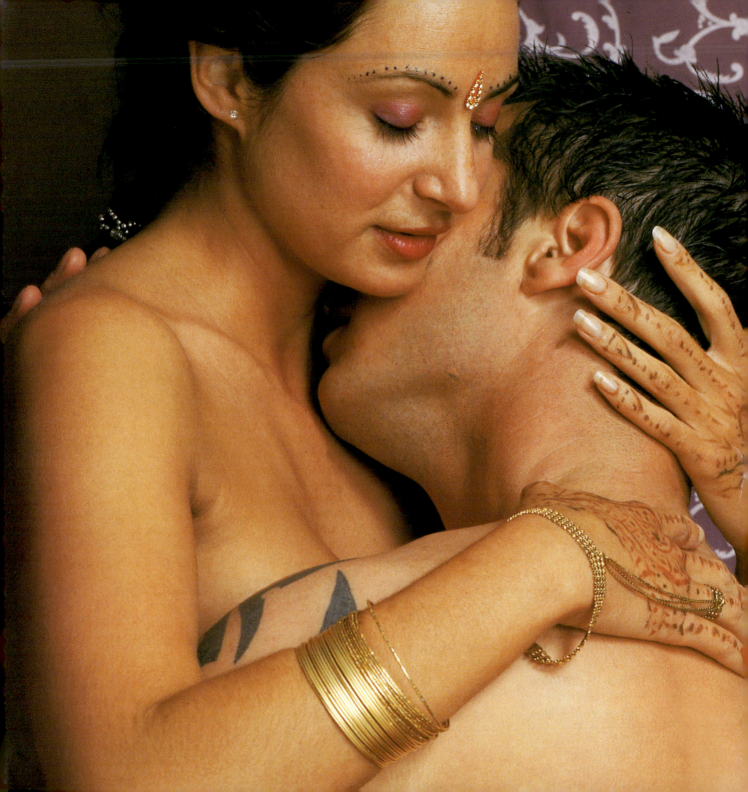

THE TEACHINGS OF THE KAMA SUTRA

Kama is enjoyment by the five senses of hearing, feeling, seeing, tasting, smelling, assisted by the mind together with the soul.

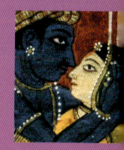

The Kama Sutra is a celebration of sensuality in all its forms. For the author, Vatsyayana, the body is a 'pleasure garden of sensual delights'. The pursuit of pleasure is not an indulgence, but part of what it means to be a well-rounded citizen. 'Pleasures,' he said, 'being as necessary for the existence and well-being of the body as food.' The Kama Sutra covers all aspects of sexual relationships, from choosing, attracting, courting and seducing a lover, to the art of lovemaking itself. The sage offers comprehensive advice. Nothing is omitted, including the role of romance, the joy of sexually arousing ointments and massage, the exquisite delights of petting and foreplay, oral and manual stimulation, sexual positions and tips to sustain lovemaking. Much of his advice, from centuries ago, is still relevant.

In Vatsyayana's day, lovemaking was also regarded as a spiritual experience. The sexual union of the male and female gods Shiva and Shakti brought the Earth into being. Therefore lovemaking enabled couples to attain a higher spiritual plane – a state of oneness more complete than anything people can achieve individually. This is the basis of Tantra, a movement influenced by Vatsyayana's teachings.

RIGHT
The body is packed with pleasure zones: it takes time to explore them all.

BELOW
A willing lover can help you discover novel areas of erotic sensitivity, and the best ways to set them tingling.

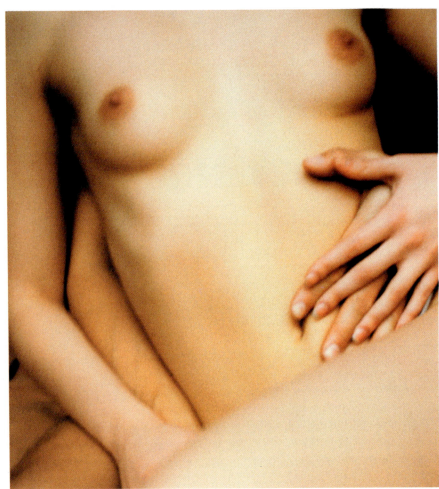

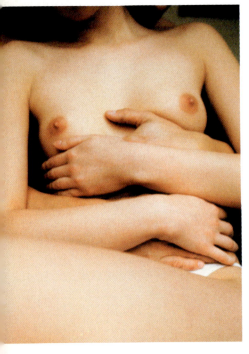

Vatsyayana regarded comprehensive sexual knowledge as vital for men and women. Young women, he said, should study the Kama Sutra before finding a partner, and continue to refer to it long afterwards. The Kama Sutra places equal emphasis on mutual pleasure. This is in contrast to the prim Victorian world into which the work's first English translator, Sir Richard Burton, was born. At that time, and for many decades afterwards, the notion that women could – and should – enjoy sex was regarded as shocking. Couples entered marriage in a state of sexual ignorance, often needing a doctor to explain the basic facts of life.

Until recent times, the sexual pose most Western couples adopted was the traditional 'missionary position', with the man lying on top of his partner with his body between her thighs. The term 'missionary position' was coined by the sexually liberated natives of the Polynesian Islands and described the only position European missionaries knew. The Polynesians themselves knew lots of ways to make love. Their favourite involved the woman sitting astride her partner, and you will find this position – and many others – described on the following pages.

THE SEXUAL BODY

For fully satisfying lovemaking, it helps to discover everything you can about your own sexual nature, and that of your partner. 'Sexual body' doesn't just mean the sex organs, or other highly sexually charged ('erogenous') zones, such as the breasts and thighs. It refers to all parts of the body, including ears, neck, back, legs and arms, which, when stimulated, evoke powerfully arousing sensations. To enjoy a total sexual experience, as Vatsyayana commended, a first step is to explore your own body, to find new areas of response and unique forms of stimulation, and to relay this knowledge to your partner.

*Men and women,
being of the same nature,
feel the same kind
of pleasure.*

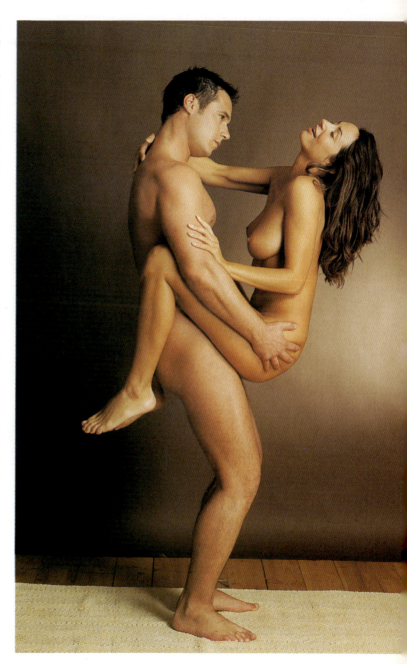

THE FEMALE SEX ORGANS

In the Kama Sutra, the term *yoni* refers to the external female genitals, or vulva, and the vagina. A woman's sex organs are more complicated than a man's so her partner, with her help, needs time to explore them and discover where and how to stimulate them. But

The vulva is the region between the pubic mound *(mons pubis)*, at the base of the abdomen, to the perineum, the soft strip of skin between vulva and anus. The vulva is covered by a pair of fleshy lips, the outer labia *(labia majora)*, which enclose the more delicate inner lips *(labia minora)*. The inner lips enclose the vestibule, a moist, pink region that includes the urethra, through which urine passes out

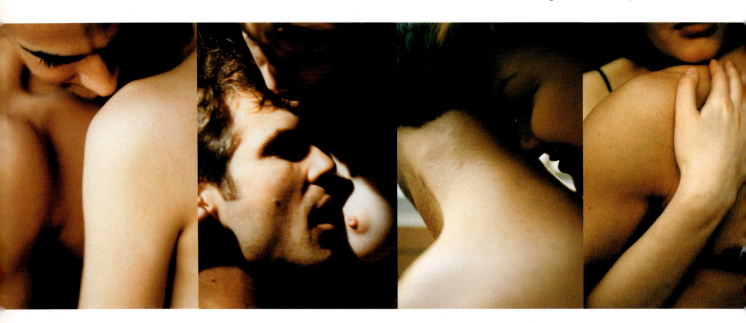

before a woman can teach her lover she must learn about them herself. Some women are reluctant to explore their vulva and vagina, perhaps from guilt or embarrassment. Once a woman can overcome such feelings, becoming more relaxed about touching herself, she'll feel more confident about guiding her partner. The best way is to study your body, using a mirror as necessary, and experimenting with where and how you like being touched. You can then encourage your partner to do the same.

of the body, and the vaginal opening. Some woman may feel self-conscious about the vulva, thinking this part of their body unattractive. Few men would agree.

ABOVE
By varying your caress and the areas of the body being stroked, you help your lover reach new heights of ecstasy.

FAR RIGHT
Teasing touches with lips and fingertips let a partner's passion slowly build up to an earth-shaking climax.

FEMALE EROGENOUS ZONES

In fact, a woman's vulva has been compared to the petals of a bloom. The multimillionaire Howard Hughes called his mistress 'Rosebud' because of this resemblance with the flower.

The most sexually sensitive part is the clitoris, located where the *labia minora* join at the front. The tip of the clitoris is usually covered by a fold of skin – the clitoral hood. When a woman becomes aroused, the clitoris swells and its tip may become visible. This tiny organ is part of a much larger internal structure. For some women, the clitoris is too sensitive to touch directly and they can tolerate only indirect stimulation over or alongside the hood. All parts of the vulva are highly sensitive, as is the outer third and rim of the vagina. But women may find the lower inner wall of the vagina, a part that tends to receive most stimulation during penetration, is not very sensitive. Intercourse alone may be insufficient to trigger orgasm and manual stimulation may be needed.

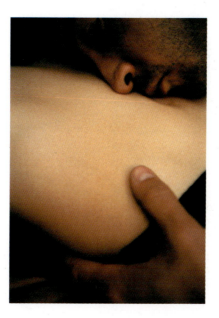

Apart from the sex organs, the most highly charged areas of a woman's body are her breasts, nipples and the darkly pigmented areas *(areolae)* that surround them, lower abdomen, especially the pubic mound, inner thigh, perineum and buttocks. But almost any part of a woman's body is a potential erogenous zone. For example, some women are powerfully turned on by having the neck or ears caressed. A woman's skin is softer and more sensitive than a man's and responds readily to a gentle touch. Her partner can experiment with delicate brushing strokes, circular movements and varying levels of pressure, to discover the kind of stimulation she likes. This is not an academic exercise: men should relish touching their partners just as much as women enjoy being touched.

SEXUAL FOCUS

The orgasm may seem an automatic response but, in fact, it has to be learned. As sexual arousal builds we need to focus inwardly on a particular area of sensation, usually the genitals, in order to reach a peak and climax. This is easier for a man because his erect penis is an obvious point of focus for his sexual feelings. But a woman has many erogenous zones – nipples, labia, clitoris, vagina – all competing for attention.

This variety of erogenous zones generates an 'all-over' pleasurable sensation that may not trigger full orgasm unless her feelings coalesce on a specific area. Some women find clitoral orgasms the most powerful, while others report that the vaginal climax is more satisfying. Whichever one is best for you is learned through self-discovery, ideally aided by a patient and imaginative lover.

THE MALE SEX ORGANS

A man's external sex organs comprise the penis and testicles. Men also have an internal prostate gland, which produces seminal fluid. This can be stimulated indirectly via the anus using, for example, a vibrator (see also pages 109–10). The testicles are covered by a sac of skin called the scrotum, or scrotal sac. When a man is aroused, his penis engorges with blood, grows longer and hardens. Vatsyayana calls the penis the 'lingam'. Penis size was an important part of Vatsyayana's studies. He classifies males as 'hare', 'bull', or 'horse' according to the length of the erect 'lingam'. This issue still troubles many males today. Yet a man's ability to satisfy a woman is not determined by penis length. Experiment, and whatever your size and shape you'll find a position that works. As only the first third of the vagina is sexually sensitive, an erect penis of almost any size can apply enough stimulation. In general, the smaller a penis when flaccid (non-aroused), the greater its size when erect – often many times larger than its relaxed state.

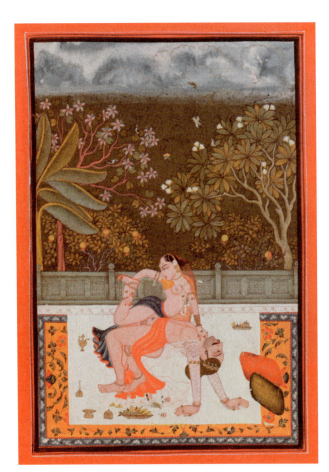

All parts of the penis are sensitive, especially when erect, but the most sensitive part is the head *(glans)*. In uncircumcised men the glans is covered by a tubular flap of skin – the foreskin. This rolls back during intercourse to expose the glans. The degree of sensitivity varies between individuals. For some men, the glans is too sensitive to touch directly, especially during manual stimulation, unless lubricating gel is used and friction is mainly applied to the shaft. The scrotal sac is also highly sensitive. Many men enjoy having the scrotum stroked and fondled during lovemaking. Males also differ in how they like to be touched. Some enjoy firm, vigorous stimulation; others less so. The best way to find out what turns a man on is by experiment. Or his partner could watch while he stimulates himself.

MALE EROGENOUS ZONES

Men have many potential erogenous zones. But as sexual stimulation in males tends to focus on the genitals, other areas receive less attention, which means men may not get as much out of lovemaking as they could. Focusing solely on genital stimulation can lead to rapid arousal and ejaculation. Ejaculating too soon, before a lover is close to orgasm, can be a source of frustration for both partners, and even harms relationships.

Making sex a total sensory experience involving all areas of the body helps men to get more out of lovemaking and control and extend their arousal, and so delay ejaculation.

The buttock cheeks and anus are among the most sexually sensitive non-genital areas. Stroking these as an arousing prelude to lovemaking, or during intercourse itself, can enhance a man's enjoyment. A neglected area of a man's body is the perineum, which is as sensitive in men as in women. Here, a partner's light touch on the delicate skin can trigger sensations never experienced before. But all parts of a man's skin respond to a delicate touch, especially when accompanied by soft, sexy words and gentle kisses. Areas well supplied with sensitive nerve endings are the neck, ears, chest, nipples, stomach and thighs.

At the first time of sexual union the male's passion is intense, and his time is short. In subsequent unions on the same day the reverse is the case.

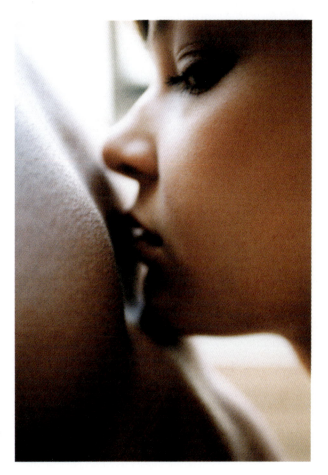

ABOVE
A man will respond powerfully to a woman's soft embrace. By concentrating on neglected areas of his body, such as his chest, she can prolong his pleasure.

FROM AROUSAL TO ORGASM

During sex both men and women pass through four distinct phases: excitement, plateau, orgasm and refractory. But the time men and women spend at each phase varies greatly.

Excitement phase In this phase, the heart and breathing rates quicken and physical changes take place that allow intercourse to occur. As the man's penis grows hard and erect, the glans darkens and the scrotal sac tightens, pulling the testicles close to the body. The woman's genitals also become engorged with blood, the vagina opens slightly and the clitoris grows erect. A natural lubricating fluid is released into the vagina to aid comfortable penetration, and some may leak from the vaginal opening. In addition, a woman's breasts enlarge slightly, the nipples grow erect and the areolae darken. A characteristic skin reddening, or 'sex flush', may appear on the chest in men and women.

Plateau phase Arousal grows until both men and women enter the pre-orgasm plateau phase. A little seminal fluid (pre-ejaculate) may leak from the penis at this time. A woman's body continues to change. The first third of the vagina widens and lengthens by up to 75 per cent, while the lower part narrows, gripping the penis more tightly. The plateau phase is longer in females than in males. As a consequence, most women need at least ten minutes more stimulation in this phase than a man in order to reach orgasm. So, unless her partner can delay or extend arousal and ejaculation, he may climax before she does (see also page 19).

> *With the female, at the first time her passion is weak, and then her time long, but on subsequent occasions on the same day, her passion is intense and her time short, until her passion is satisfied.*

FAR RIGHT
Taking the more dominant, on-top position, a woman controls the pace of love-making and so ensures she gets all the sexual stimulation she needs.

SIMULTANEOUS ORGASMS

Differences in sexual response between men and women make simultaneous orgasm difficult to achieve. As long as both partners are satisfied, this need not matter. But some couples feel sex lacks emotional intimacy unless they can climax together, showing they are sexually 'in tune'. The best way to achieve simultaneous orgasm is to ensure the woman is highly aroused – and close to orgasm – before penetration, using manual stimulation, oral sex or a vibrator.

As re-arousal is slower in a man, couples may find that repeating intercourse – after a short rest – means they are more likely to climax together. Age, too, reduces the difference in a couple's sexual response as men generally take longer to climax as they get older, whereas women often find that, over time, they are aroused more easily.

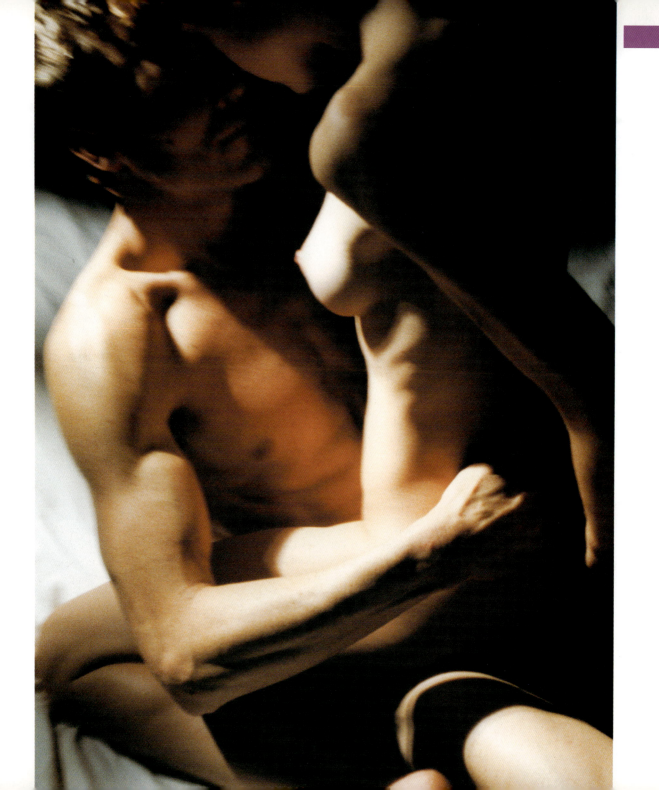

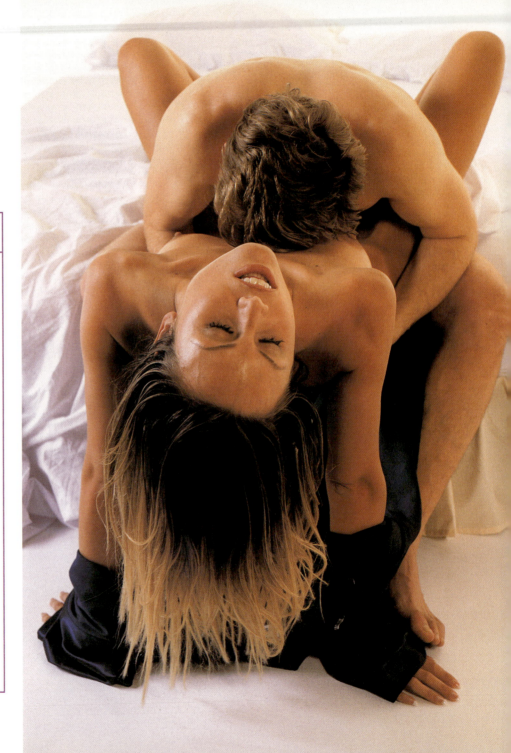

RIGHT
By varying techniques and positions, couples can find a method of lovemaking to suit them both.

THE G-SPOT

One area of the vagina is highly sexually sensitive. This is the G-spot (full name, the 'Grafenburg spot', named after the gynaecologist who first identified it). It is located on the front wall of the vagina, about 5 cm (2 in) from the entrance. When stimulated, it swells to form a small lump that is sensitive enough to bring a woman to orgasm. It can be difficult to find, and reach, except manually, or with the aid of a vibrator or other sex toy.

Some positions described in the book help bring the penis into contact with the G-spot, but individual anatomy and flexibility vary, so practise is the best way.

Orgasm phase If stimulation continues, both partners reach sexual climax. The man ejaculates, thigh muscles tense, abdominal muscles contract in waves and his toes may curl. Pleasurable orgasmic feelings can last 15–20 seconds, before subsiding. A woman's orgasm lasts longer: 20–30 seconds on average. Waves of rhythmic contractions spread through her sexual organs, her lower abdomen and thighs tense up and her back may arch. In both sexes, the sex flush may darken and spread over the body. As they climax men and women may gasp or cry out, or simply remain quiet. Some women laugh or even cry because of the sudden release of sexual tension.

Refractory phase This is the winding-down stage when the body reverts to its pre-arousal state. It is felt as a period of relaxation and fatigue. Men, in particular, may feel sleepy. For young men, resolution can last a matter of minutes only, but with age this phase lengthens, and older men must let several hours elapse before re-arousal. In contrast to the plateau phase, resolution is shorter in females. Women stimulated soon after orgasm may re-enter plateau phase and swiftly climax. This is known as multiple orgasm.

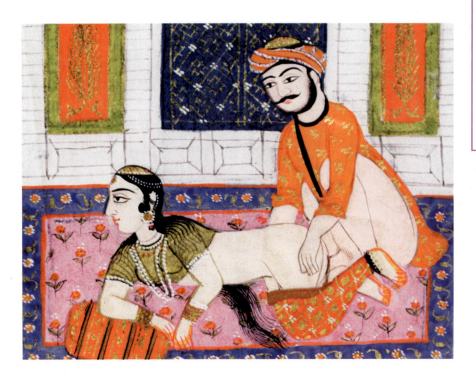

DELAYING EJACULATION

A man can delay ejaculation by slowing his thrusting movements and tightening his pelvic floor muscles (see page 24). Thinking unsexy thoughts helps too. Alternatively, he can withdraw completely and stimulate his partner manually until she nears climax, and then continue with intercourse.

Another method, the 'squeeze technique', is useful for men prone to premature ejaculation. Here, the man withdraws and then he or his partner grips the penis just under the glans for a few seconds until the erection begins to subside. Then penetration resumes. This is repeated two or three times until his partner approaches orgasm and he can carry on until they climax.

As dough is prepared for baking, so must a woman be prepared for sexual intercourse, if she is to derive satisfaction from it.

THE SEXUAL MIND

Men and women have a different mental approach to sex. A woman's self-image and feelings about her partner greatly affect how easily she gets aroused. Couples are most highly sexually charged early on in a relationship. Romance and emotional rapport play a major part in a woman's sexual feelings. In fact, love can be the strongest aphrodisiac of all and may keep her libido strong for as long as she feels good about the relationship and is enjoying regular, loving sex. For men, however, having a new partner – and a new body to explore – is the main stimulus. The way his new lover looks and feels, how she dresses, her unique scent (natural, rather than bottled) and her voice are powerful stimulants. To continue to be aroused by a partner, a man may need variety in lovemaking, such as change of positions, sexy clothing or sex toys (see pages 41, 109–10). Plenty of ideas for spicing up sex can be found throughout the book.

In women, sexual arousal varies according to the time of the day or day of the month. Women may find their libido strongest around the mid-point in their menstrual cycle, at the time of ovulation, or just before or after menstruation. Other factors that affect a couple's desire for lovemaking include age, illness, overwork, stress and emotional difficulties, such as trying for a baby. Many of these problems can be overcome through communication, simply by talking over the issues and perhaps by adapting lovemaking. For example, a sensual massage (see pages 46–9) can ease tension and stress, and prepare partners for lovemaking. Side-by-side positions (see pages 84–5) are less strenuous and encourage tender, loving, more emotionally enriching sex. The woman-on-top position (see pages 82–3) adds spice to a sexual relationship, and shares the physical demands of lovemaking.

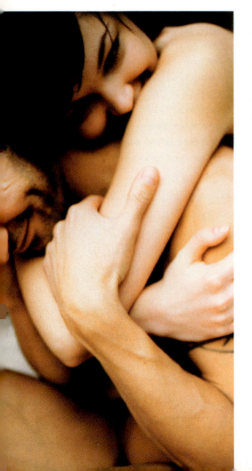

BELOW
How a woman feels about her man and the state of their relationship determines how much pleasure she gets from sex with him.

*Men who are acquainted
with the act of love are well aware
how often one woman
differs from another in her sighs and
sounds during the time of congress.*

THE SEXUAL MIND

EROTIC PATHWAY

The psychologist David Reed identified four psychological stages of sexual response: seduction, sensation, surrender and reflection. These form a kind of erotic mental pathway. 'Seduction' is the sexual attraction that triggers arousal. 'Sensation' is the stage at which the senses – sight, sound, smell, touch and taste – are stimulated during arousal, bombarding the brain with sexual signals. 'Surrender' is mental and emotional release, allowing climax to occur. In the postorgasm 'reflection' stage, couples evaluate the lovemaking that took place, mentally awarding positive marks, which help strengthen the relationship, or negative marks, which may weaken it. Emotions such as stress, fear or anger block this pathway. Just before climaxing, men enter a stage of 'ejaculatory inevitability' when orgasm cannot be prevented. But a woman can be distracted by a sound, word or thought right up to the moment of climax and may then lose interest in lovemaking.

BELOW
Taking time to lie folded in each other's arms, as you bask in postcoital bliss, will intensify your love for one another.

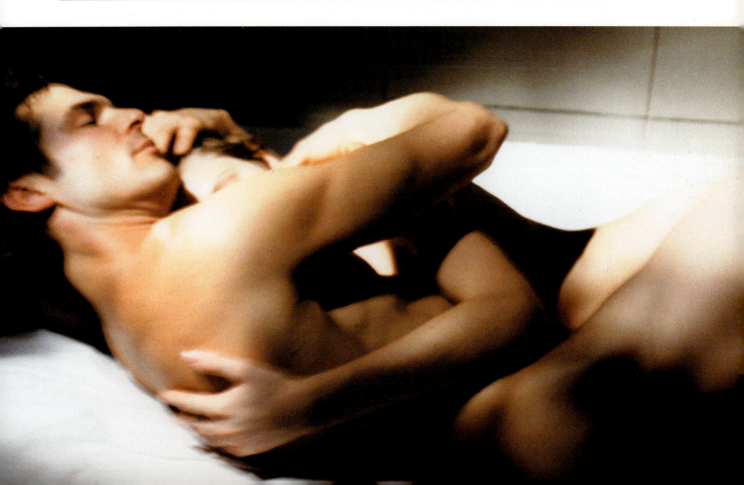

THE HEALTHY BODY

BELOW
Pelvic squats and (far right) pelvic circles can increase your range of movement so you can enjoy adventurous sex.

You don't need to be a highly trained athlete or flexible gymnast to enjoy sex, though sex is a very physical activity. It requires stamina and may involve positions not encountered at other times. Vatsyayana encouraged followers to seek physical improvement. A well-planned exercise programme enhances lovemaking. Aerobic exercise such as brisk walking, jogging, swimming or cycling improves stamina, enabling you to be sexually energetic without

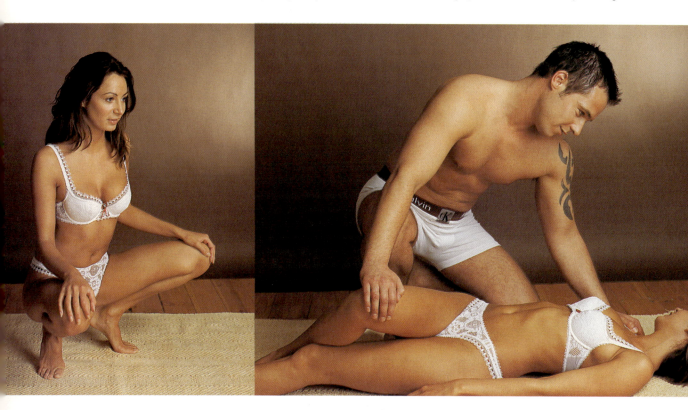

ABOVE RIGHT
Combined exercises such as the partner-aided stretch brings you both together as a couple.

becoming breathless or fatigued. Flexibility exercise aids suppleness so you can achieve more adventurous positions. Muscle-strengthening exercise allows you to hold positions for longer without cramp curbing your passion. Some muscles and joints have to work especially hard during sex: hips, thighs and lower back are particularly important. The following exercises may help.

Pelvic circles Stand facing forward with your feet shoulder-width apart. Place your hands on your hips and move your pelvis in wide circles, six times clockwise and six times anticlockwise, inhaling and exhaling smoothly and evenly.

Squats Stand with the feet shoulder-width apart. Slowly squat down as low as is comfortable. If you wish, hold on to a chair for support. Stay squatting for a count of five and then stand. Repeat two or three times.

Inner-thigh stretch Sit on the floor with the soles together and knees pointing out to the sides. Pull your ankles as close to you as is comfortable.

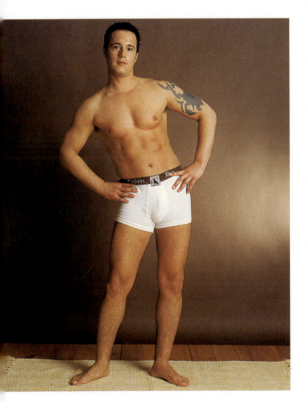

Using your elbows, press your knees down towards the floor as far as is comfortable and, at the same time, resist the downward pressure by pushing up with the legs. You should feel your inner-thigh muscles tightening. Hold for a count of ten. Repeat two or three times.

Knees to chest Lie on your back and draw your knees up towards your chest. Place your hands on your knees. Inhale, pushing your knees away from you until your arms are straight. Exhale, drawing the knees back towards your body. Repeat two or three times.

Partner-aided hip stretch By exercising together, you enhance intimacy in a relationship. In this exercise, you and your partner take turns to assist each other in a stretch. Lie on your back with your shoulders flat on the floor. Raise your right knee and let it drop to the left side. Keeping your shoulders flat, turn your face to the right. Your partner kneels by your right side and places one hand on your right shoulder and the other on your right knee and gently presses down as far as is comfortable for you. Repeat on the other side. Now change places.

Bathe daily, using a lathering substance, applying ointments and perfumes to the body, placing ornaments on the person, and applying colour to the lips. All these things should be done without fail.

PELVIC FLOOR

The pelvic floor comprises muscles, ligaments and other tissues that support the bladder, urethra and rectum in men and women, and the vagina and uterus in women. To find your pelvic floor, imagine you need to urinate but must hold back. To do this, tighten the pelvic floor muscles (also called 'love muscles', because of their role in sex). By strengthening the pelvic floor, a woman can grip her partner's penis more firmly, increasing the pleasurable sensations they both feel. The man can tighten his pelvic floor to slow his own arousal, if he is climaxing too soon. Tantrikas – experts in tantric sex (see pages 111–3) – call these fire muscles, as they are regarded as a source of sexual energy, spreading through the lower body like flames. They are important in Tantric sex to delay orgasm, and so increase sexual and spiritual energy.

The following pelvic exercises (also called Kegel exercises) strengthen the pelvic floor. Aim to do them several times a day, wherever you are: sitting in your car or on a train, watching TV or waiting for water to boil. No one can see you do them. To start, sit on a firm seat, with legs slightly apart. Breathing normally, draw up your pelvic floor. Hold for ten seconds and then slowly relax. Pelvic floor muscles tire quickly, so do only a few repetitions at first. As you get stronger, increase them up to a maximum of ten.

Another method is to tighten the pelvic floor muscles and then immediately let go. Do up to ten of these at a time. To check whether you are doing the exercises effectively, next time you urinate, try to slow or stop the flow of urine, but don't do this too often as the increased pressure puts a strain on the kidneys.

You can combine Kegel exercises with pelvic squats. Place the feet hip-width apart and squat down, holding on to your feet for support. Relax your pelvic floor. Take five short in-breaths, steadily tightening your pelvic floor with each breath. Now give five short out-breaths, steadily relaxing your pelvic floor as you do so. Repeat this up to ten times.

SEXUAL HYGIENE

The Kama Sutra devotes much space to cleansing, especially as a prelude to lovemaking. Vatsyayana's message is as relevant now as it was in his day. Feeling fresh and clean helps builds self-confidence during intimate moments with a lover. But it is not necessary to remove or mask all natural aromas. Fresh

---

FAR RIGHT
By showering together at the end of a hectic day, you benefit from the relaxing effect of the soothing cascade, and the really fresh feeling.

SEX DURING MENSTRUATION

The issue of whether or not to make love during a woman's period is obviously a highly personal one. Some religions forbid the practice, but otherwise, provided both partners feel comfortable about it, there is no reason not to have sex at this time. However, there is still a risk of pregnancy, so using a barrier contraception, such as a condom, is important.

SEXUAL HYGIENE   25

sweat has no smell so a daily bath, shower or all-over wash is all that is necessary to stay smelling sweet.

A woman may be self-conscious about her natural scent and wonder how a man may react to it. She need have no fears. Far from being a sexual turn-off, a woman's unique aroma acts as an aphrodisiac, changing over the course of her menstrual cycle, becoming faintly 'musky' as she approaches ovulation, when she is at her most fertile. The bodies of both sexes also release pheromones – odourless sexual attractants that can entice a mate.

Sexual hygiene for men and women means paying attention to the anal and pubic zones. Uncircumcised men should ensure the area underneath the foreskin is kept clean. An oily secretion, called smegma, is produced here. It acts as a lubricant, allowing the foreskin to move freely over the glans. Unless care is taken, smegma builds up and can harbour infection. For a woman, simple bathing is sufficient to keep the vulva cleansed. Highly scented vaginal soaps, douches or deodorants should be avoided as this area is self-cleansing. Such chemicals can upset the vagina's delicate bacterial balance, leading to irritation and inflammation. It is important to wash the anal area from front to back to avoid transferring infectious micro-organisms to the vagina.

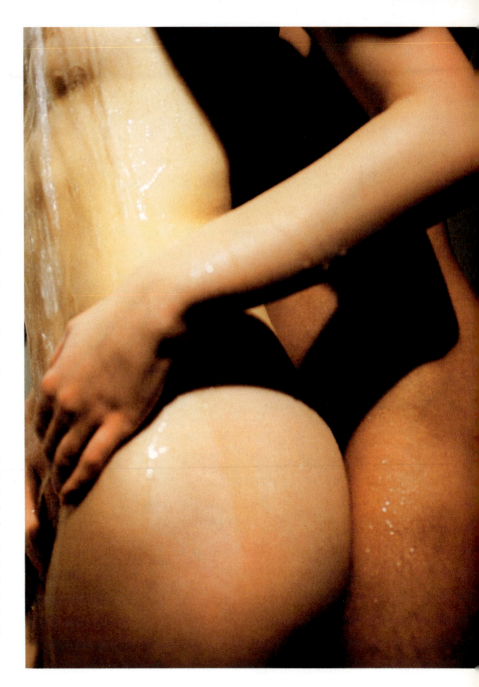

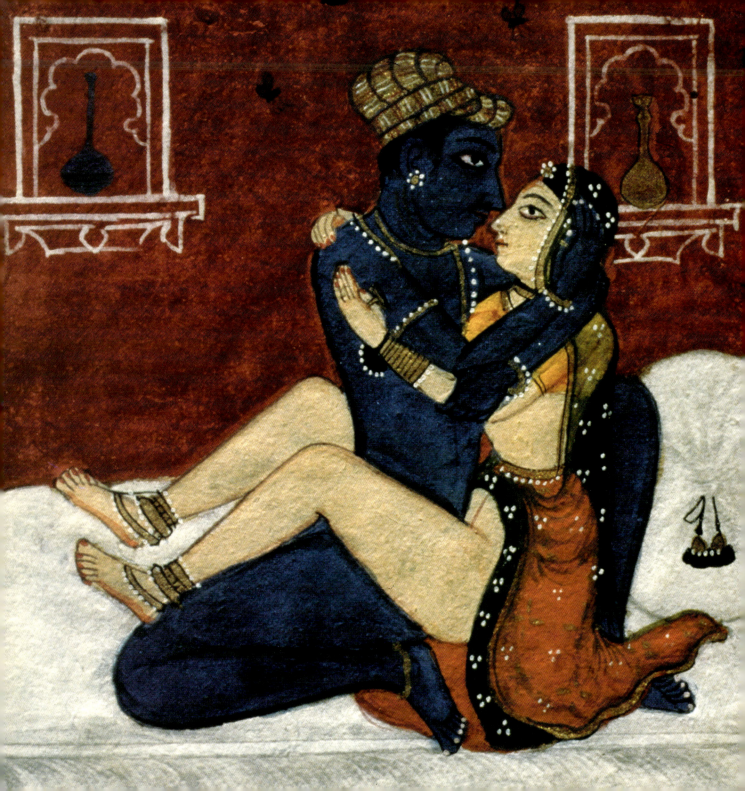

THE SENSUAL BODY

The importance of stimulating all the senses, of bringing sensuality into everything you do, is a cornerstone of the Kama Sutra. Vatsyayana encourages lovers to make full use of oils, fragrances, sounds and massage to enhance romance. Aromas released from an oil burner to scent the air, or added to the bath water, stimulate the olfactory sense, which has a direct line to the primitive limbic system of the brain. Music, softly playing in the background, evokes a romantic mood. But no sound is as sensual as the voice so never miss a chance to talk to your lover softly. This is called 'whispering sweet nothings', as the words matter less than the tone and emotion revealed.

BELOW LEFT

Men and women are strongly aroused by the groans and gasps of passion a lover emits at the height of ecstasy.

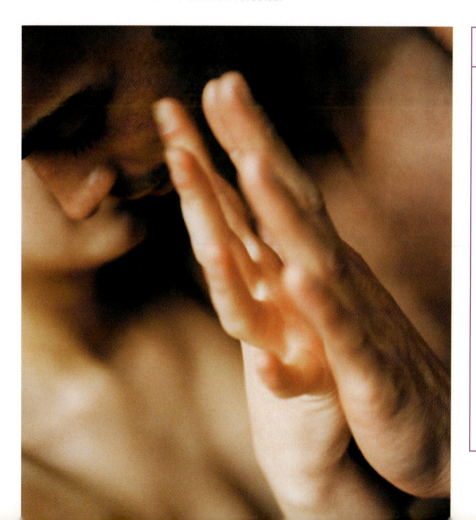

SEX SOUNDS

The voice is an amazing sexual tool – both in its sound and in language. Both sexes, and men in particular, are powerfully aroused by a partner's sexy words. Some men are turned on by erotic language – hence the popularity of telephone sex lines.

Women often find that 'vocalizing' their feelings during sex helps them to climax. And the husky tone, groans, gasps and other sounds women may make when approaching orgasm heighten a man's sexual arousal – and he knows he's getting it right!

THE SENSUAL SKIN

FAR RIGHT
Moistening a nipple with your tongue and then gently blowing across it, can arouse mind-tingling sensations in your partner.

The sense of touch is particularly acute yet we may be unaware of the full range of tactile sensations we can experience. All parts of the skin are packed with nerve endings, each responding to distinct stimuli, such as light touch, firm pressure, heat, cold, vibration and stretch. A woman's skin is softer than a man's, which may be why women derive more pleasure from tactile stimulation. Taking time together to explore this sense, the different ways of touching and places to be touched brings a new dimension to a relationship. The aim is not to arouse a partner but to discover all the highly pleasurable sensations that simple skin contact can offer. See how lightly you can touch the skin and still get a response, tracing the contours of face and neck, or teasingly across the inner thigh. The type and arrangement of nerve endings varies over the body, so try different strokes for different areas, altering pressure to see how your partner's body responds. Use the back of the fingers, too, or stroke the skin gently with the nails.

When you have experimented with feather-light touches, try a feather itself. In Vatsyayana's exotic eastern world, the ultimate sensory tool was a plume plucked from a peacock or ostrich, lovingly stroked over breast and along thigh. But any feather works well. Try other materials, such as different fabrics: caress the skin with silk, satin or chiffon. If you have long hair, sweep it back and forth over your partner's body.

Experiment with different temperatures, such as ice, a warm shower spray, or melted chocolate. These stimulate a different set of nerves, arousing new sensations. Run the ice cube over the chest, between the breasts, or over the flat of the stomach. Or hold it in your mouth and apply it to the back or legs. (For additional sensual ideas, see pages 96–113.) The tongue stimulates a wide range of experiences, lightly flicking the skin with its tip, or following curves of ears and neck, bathing the surface with deliciously moist sensations.

SENSUAL BREATH

Blowing across the skin stimulates delicate nerve endings at the base of the hair follicles. These quiver and create a delicious tingling sensation to arouse and excite your partner. Try moistening or lubricating the skin, and then directing a gentle jet of air over the surface from your mouth, a partly inflated balloon or a small fan. Use circular movements to create mini whirlwinds. This feels particularly good over nipples, buttocks or genitals.

THE SENSUAL SKIN | 29

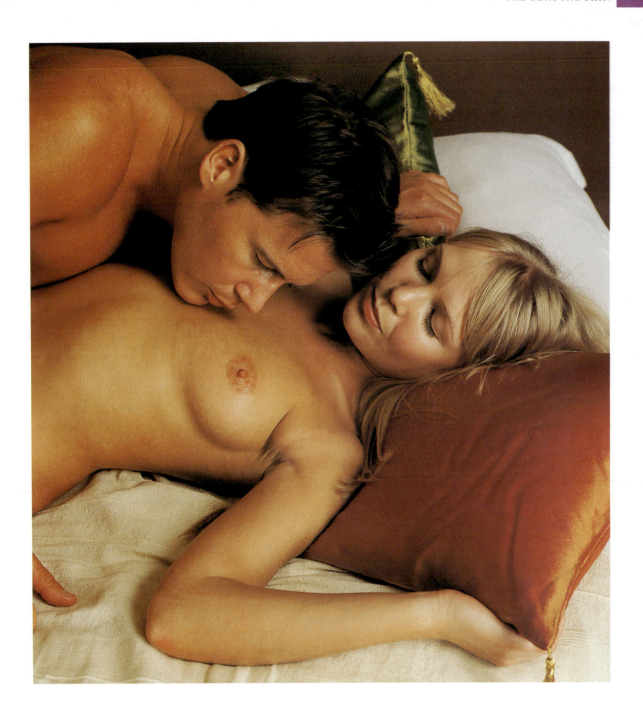

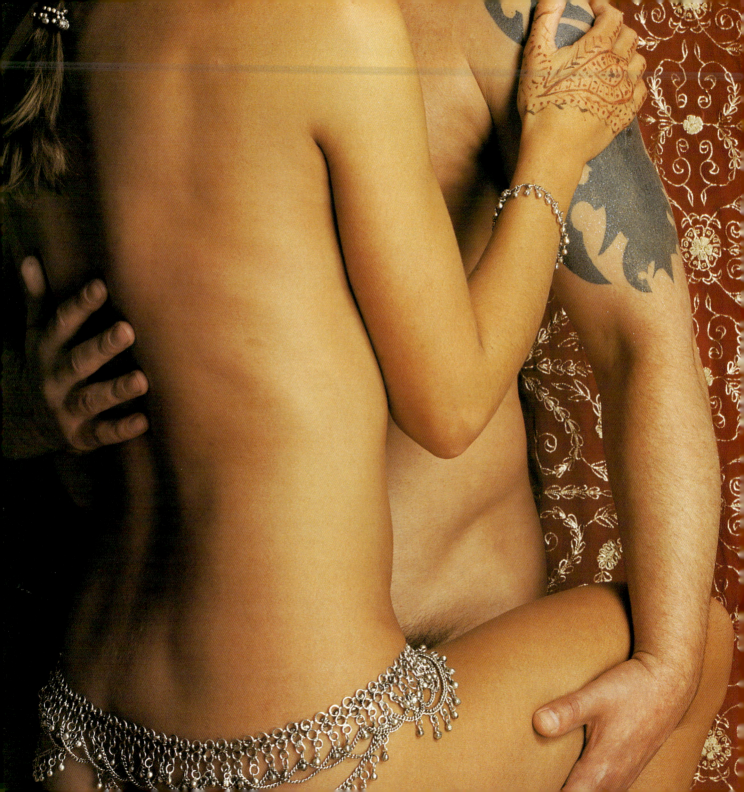

ATTRACTING A PARTNER

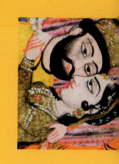

A man who has seen and perceived the feelings of the woman towards him, and who has noticed the outward signs and movements by which those feelings are expressed, should do everything in his power to effect a union.

The Kama Sutra offers advice on all aspects of romantic life, including where and how to meet potential partners. In Vatsyayana's time, society was very different but the basic principles still hold true. To find that special 'someone' you must frequent the places your kindred spirit is likely to be. It is over-optimistic to expect a soulmate to track *you* down, wherever you are. As you circulate, the way you dress, how you present yourself and what you say all project an image of the person you are – *and* the person you want to attract. You also reveal much about yourself subconsciously, through body language – the postures and subtle mannerisms that signpost your innermost thoughts.

CONFIDENCE AND SELF-KNOWLEDGE

Having confidence in yourself is an important first step in any relationship. Confidence comes from self-knowledge – knowing who you are and what you want – and self-belief – the conviction that you are what you want to be. If this seems simplistic, take your lead from Vatsyayana. He exudes self-confidence. Once attracted to someone, he plans a strategy that will bring the two of them together so that he can beguile her with his charms. And he has little doubt that he will succeed. Most of us cannot enjoy the sumptuous lifestyle of an Indian prince, but we can try to exude that same self-confidence. If this seems difficult, bear in mind that if you lack confidence in yourself, the chances are that any person you meet is feeling similarly unsure about him- or herself. Once the ice is broken and you begin to chat, you'll both wonder why you were so worried.

KAMA QUEST

First you must find that special person. Many couples meet at work, which is not surprising as it fulfils four important criteria for forming relationships. First, the workplace offers plenty of opportunities for both sexes to come into contact. Second, you have lots of things in common to talk about, such as work issues and colleagues. Third, you are probably well matched, as people of similar outlooks tend to enter similar careers. Fourth, you spend long periods of the day in close proximity, thus giving any budding romance the chance to blossom.

If there's no one at work who seems right for you, look further afield. As a prelude to courtship the Kama Sutra encourages citizens to indulge in the widest possible range of social diversions. These include riding in public gardens, mixed bathing in rivers and swimming pools, and moonlight picnics. More practically today, however, leisure and sports clubs, social groups, political affiliations and special interest societies offer golden opportunities to meet potential partners. The same rules apply as in the workplace. Choose a venue where you'll meet others with similar interests, and where you can start a conversation and talk easily. Ensure it is something you really enjoy, and will want to keep doing. A budding relationship has little hope of success if you find yourself doing something you loathe, surrounded by those who can talk of little else, just to find a partner.

> *He who knows how to make himself beloved by women, as well as to increase their honour and create confidence in them, this man becomes an object of their love.*

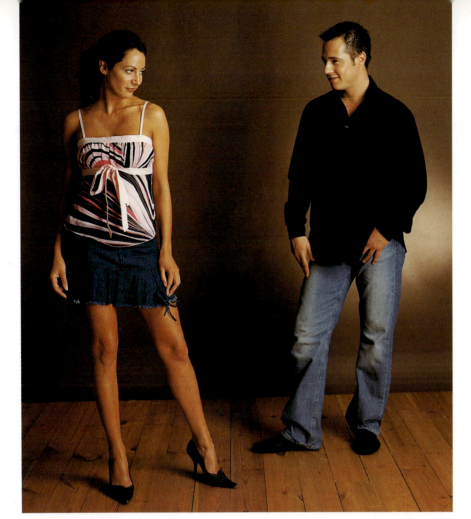

LEFT
The signs that a woman is interested in a man are subtle – often little more than a brief glance and a change of stance.

THE SIXTY-FOUR ARTS

Vatsyayana knew that sexual attraction alone could not sustain a relationship. There also needed to be *'the power to attract the minds of others'*. In the Kama Sutra, cultivated men and women were advised to acquaint themselves with the *'sixty-four arts'*. Vatsyayana did not expect individuals to be expert in every one of them, but to be proficient in around ten, and to know something of the others. This allowed them to talk knowledgeably and on equal terms with potential lovers. The range of subjects listed in the Kama Sutra is vast and includes literature, art, dance, music, science, gardening and sport. Women, it says, who are *'versed in the above arts ... become objects of universal regard'*.

KAMA COURTSHIP

How can you tell if anyone you meet feels the same way about you? Vatsyayana knew that women do not just leave it to the man to initiate a relationship, for he describes as *'idle talk'* a belief that women *'make no effort themselves to gain over the object of their affections'*. But he also knew the signals of attraction that women emit are subtle. A woman *'never looks the man in the face'* but *'looks secretly at him though he has gone away from her side'* and speaks in a way that *'attracts his attention towards her when she is at a distance from him'*. Of course women are more assertive today than in Vatsyayana's era, but they may still be reluctant to make an overt first move, at least until they have good reason to believe the object of their desire feels the same way. It is body language that reveals a couple's hidden feelings for one another.

Psychologists say that up to 65 per cent of face-to-face communication is non-verbal. Women are generally better than men at picking up these subtle clues especially when watching other couples. Repeated eye contact is an initial sign of attraction, glancing just long enough to catch the other person's eye, then looking away again. Men and women also unconsciously hold themselves straighter and taller when they think they are being observed. The two people then steadily reduce the distance between them until they are close enough to strike up a conversation. They may brush against each other, or subtly touch hands or arms. A smile of welcome is a good sign, so long as it involves the eyes, as indicated by the 'smile lines' that form in the corners. Two people who are attracted to each other may subconsciously position themselves to block out all other members of the group, so that they have each other's exclusive attention.

One of them will make a comment or ask a question, intended to break the ice. The remark may seem inane, or pointless – we can't all be Oscar Wilde, especially when nervous – but this is an opening gambit only. The aim now is to keep the talk flowing, until the subject can be steered round to something you both feel comfortable with. Once a couple begin to get acquainted, there are two types of non-verbal sign that show powerful emotions are stirring – and that the feeling is mutual. These are known as 'displacement activities' and 'mirroring' (see opposite).

> *Whenever he gives anything to her or takes anything from her, he should show by his manner and look how much he loves her ... he should express his love to her more by manner and signs than by words.*

> *The man should begin to win her over, and to create confidence in her, but should abstain at first from sexual pleasures. Women, being of a tender nature, want tender beginnings.*

LOVE
SIGNALS

Strong feelings of sexual attraction affect the primitive emotional centres of the brain such as the limbic system, over which we have little control. Hormones are released that cause physical changes such as a rise in heart and breathing rates, and increased sweating. Our animal ancestors felt no need to hide their emotions. But social conditioning forces modern humans to remain cool, calm and collected.

The conflict is resolved by a form of behaviour called 'displacement activity', such as smoothing down the clothes. A woman may pat her hair or lick her lips. A man may adjust his tie or fidget with his cuffs. Other signs include nervous giggles or hurried, garbled (and often incoherent) speech – the 'blurts'. As a couple become more friendly, another form of behaviour – 'mirroring' – occurs. They unconsciously copy each other's posture and movements, leaning forwards or backwards at the same time, sitting or standing at the same angle to each other, and simultaneously sipping from their drinks. As the relationship grows more intimate, the mirroring actions synchronize more closely.

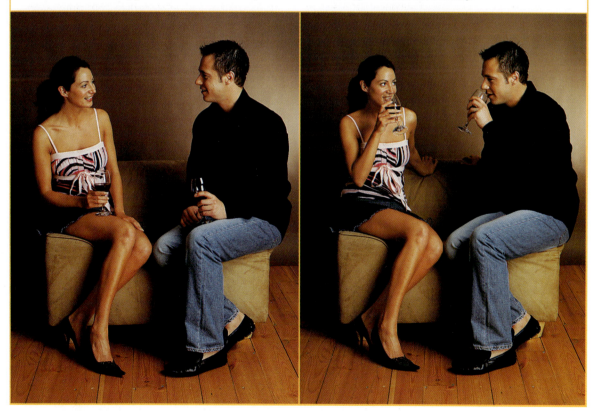

THE DATING GAME

The next step is to arrange a formal date. Ideally, choose a location that allows you to be on your own together and to talk freely without being disturbed. After all, you still have a great deal to find out about each other. Bars and restaurants are popular choices. Avoid meeting in the cinema or at a sports event the first time, though, unless planning to have a meal or drink afterwards, as there will be too many distractions to talk freely. After two or three more dates you'll know whether the initial spark is growing into a raging inferno. You'll soon want to move the relationship on to the next stage, by bringing your partner back to your home for a romantic evening. For Vatsyayana, setting the mood, seduction and foreplay were arts well worth cultivating.

THE ATMOSPHERE FOR ROMANCE

Creating a romantic mood is an essential preliminary to an intimate evening – or night – together. This is true not only for couples in the early stages of a relationship, but also for those who have been sexual partners for many years. For women, in particular, a romantic build-up strengthens the emotional bond that is a vital prelude to a night of passion. There is little hope of sexual chemistry developing unless a woman feels some empathy with her partner. Ambience is even more important if work or family problems are weighing heavily on her mind. Men, too, may find that the right atmosphere helps stir sensual feelings after a stress-filled day in the office.

Whether you opt for dinner at a cosy restaurant or a candle-lit supper at home, a romantic meal sets the emotional tone for the evening and allows more senses – smell and taste – to be stimulated. Presentation is important, as the pleasure of eating is enhanced by an attractively arranged table. This is something men must bear in mind if they host the evening. Any man who knows how to produce a tasty, attractively arranged meal for his lover will always win points. If his partner is preparing the food, the man should help – for example, by setting the table, pouring the wine, and selecting the music. Choose something light to eat; a heavy meal encourages sleepiness. A menu offering a variety of subtle flavours is best. Some foods such as oysters are known for stimulating sexual desire, but avoid highly spiced foods or dominant flavours like garlic.

THE ATMOSPHERE FOR ROMANCE   37

APHRODISIAC FOODS

Vatsyayana not only considered that delicious foods set the mood for intimacy, he also believed that energy foods (such as milk, liquorice, honey and sugar) and spicy foods (such as ginger and peppers) can fuel and inflame sexual feelings.

A firm favourite, described in the Kama Sutra and still popular today, is asparagus dipped in butter. The sexual symbolism of slipping succulent spears of asparagus into a lover's mouth is clear.

Many 'love foods' with an ancient history are now known to contain chemicals that stimulate desire. These include almonds, ginger, cinnamon and ginseng, long regarded in the East as aids to romance. The spices were often made into sweetmeats and given as love tokens. Oysters are rich in zinc, a mineral necessary for fertility. Chocolate contains energy-boosting sugar and is packed with mood-enhancing chemicals. Bananas are not only energy-rich but contain alkaloids that act on neurotransmitters (brain signalling molecules) to stimulate relaxation and contentment.

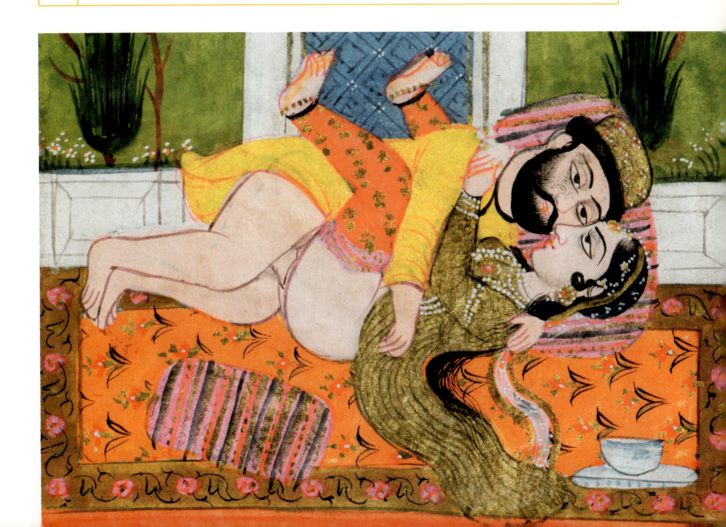

The best-known aphrodisiac, apart from love itself, is alcohol. Vatsyayana believed that *'men and women should drink in one another's houses ... liquors such as* Madhu, Aireya, Sara *and* Asawa ... *also drinks concocted from the barks of various trees, wild fruits and leaves'*. Our choices today are less exotic. But one favourite, popular then as now, is wine. In the Kama Sutra, drinking wine in moderation is portrayed as a friendly social custom, but men should drink wine *'only after the women have been served'*. Sharing a glass or two of a light, refreshing wine is a simple and pleasant way to relax and unwind together; or for added sparkle, share a bottle of champagne. Take care not to overdo it, however. A little alcohol encourages arousal but too much inhibits performance. At the very least, drink can make you drowsy. More important still, excess alcohol encourages risky behaviour – which is not a good idea during the early stages of a relationship when you don't fully know your partner's history.

THE SENSUAL ENVIRONMENT

Vatsyayana understood the need to create an environment that appeals to all the senses in order to promote sexual harmony and allow intimacy to flower. The Kama Sutra describes the ideal room for love as *'balmy with rich perfumes'* and containing *'a bed, soft, agreeable to the sight, covered with a clean white cloth ... having garlands and bunches of flowers upon it, and a canopy above'*. Nearby there should be *'ointments for the night, as well as flowers, pots containing fragrant substances'*. Scented candles can help create that exotic Eastern atmosphere, filling the air with sensual fragrances and casting soft shadows to create an intimate ambience – your very own *'oasis of sensual pleasures'*.

All couples have their own ideas about the ideal love nest. But enhancing the sensual atmosphere allows partners to open up to their desire in a relaxed and spontaneous way. Lovemaking does not have to take place in the bedroom. If the sexual flame is kindled by lying on a rug in front of an open fire or cuddling on the couch, why not make love there? A change from the usual lovemaking location brings sweet rewards. Whether you prefer bedroom or living room, there are tips for creating a sensual environment that apply in all cases. Choose decor, fabrics and furnishings in muted designs and soft, neutral colours so you only focus on what's important – each other. Similarly, keep the room uncluttered, with space to move around, so you will not get distracted or end up with bruises from the furniture.

FAR RIGHT
There's no need to rush these first intimate moments together. The more gradual the build-up, the more intense the climax will be.

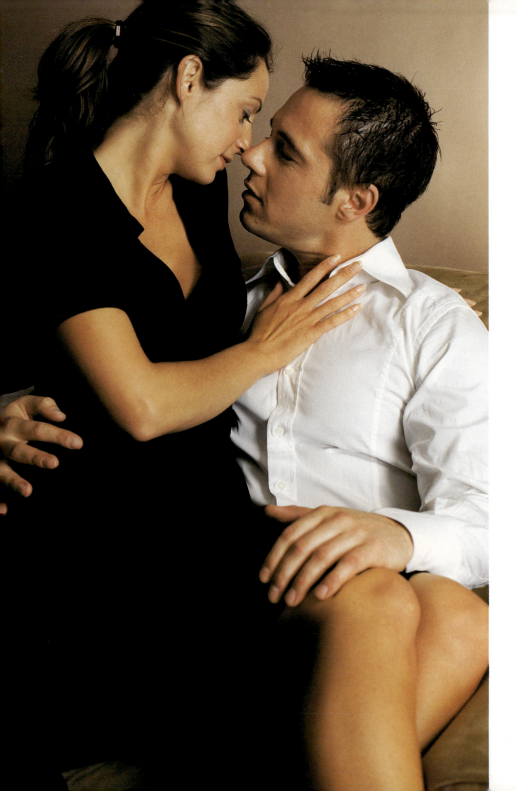

The man should therefore approach the woman according to her liking, and should make use of those devices by which he may be able to establish himself more and more into her confidence.

BELOW RIGHT
By creating a warm and sensuous environment, you encourage a relaxed mood that invites intimacy.

Keep the room feeling pleasantly warm, even after you have shed some clothing, but not too warm – things are likely to get steamy enough later on as it is – as a stuffy room can cause sleepiness. Open a window slightly to let in some air and place a small bowl of water near the radiator to humidify the room. Fresh flowers add colour and fragrance, or use exotic aromatherapy essences released from an oil burner to scent the room. Low lighting from table lamps or wall lights creates an air of mystery and allows you both to undress without feeling inhibited. Soft music completes the mood. In the living room, a deep-pile rug and a liberal scattering of cushions invites spontaneous and adventurous fun. Now you have set the scene for Kama Sutra seduction and foreplay.

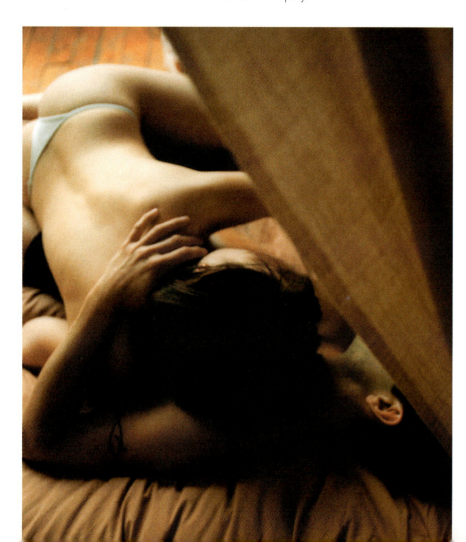

SEDUCTION AND FOREPLAY

As the evening develops, take every chance to touch each other, seemingly accidentally, and then more overtly. These brief but repeated moments of undemanding physical contact help develop and strengthen emotional ties. Remember to keep the conversation going. If you are still relative strangers, this is an important opportunity to find out a little more about each other, your likes and dislikes, and to seek out areas of interest you share. As the romantic mood takes hold, you'll be eager to demonstrate your feelings in more intimate ways. A woman responds best to a tender, attentive man who takes pains to make her feel wanted and desired. Don't feel embarrassed to say what first attracted you to your partner, what it is you like about him or her, and how much your lover turns you on. The meanings of the words now are less important than the way they are said. Terms of endearment said soft and low quickly turn to kissing and cuddles on the sofa, or on the rug or cushions you have thoughtfully placed on the floor in advance.

There is no need to rush these moments, so make them last. The longer you devote to the build-up, the more intense will be the pleasure for both of you. Stroke each other through your clothes, delighting in the feel of flesh through soft, silky material. Now you can start exploring inside each other's clothes,

SEXUAL DRESSING

Naturally, you'll want to look your best for your intimate evening. This means wearing whatever suits you and highlights your best features. But there are other points to bear in mind. Choosing loose, comfortable clothing leaves you free to move and to relax. Ideally, they should be items that you won't mind getting crumpled (it can spoil the magic of the moment if you break off to hang up a dress or trousers).

Avoid tight clothes that you must wriggle out of, or ones with awkward fastenings that you, or your partner, may struggle to undo. But don't be in too much of a hurry to strip off. The right clothes can be a powerful turn-on, so give your partner time to enjoy them. They should be roomy enough to allow wandering hands free access to explore and excite. Soft, silky natural fabrics, especially sexy underwear, feel good to touch and add to the sensual experience. Adding extra layers that a partner must remove offers more opportunities for touching and teasing and extends foreplay.

BELOW
Enjoy the feel of your lover's body through and under his or her clothes – the sensuous touch of natural fabrics can heighten the pleasure you feel.

opening zips and buttons just wide enough to allow fingers to enter and begin their voyage of discovery. A secret of foreplay is to avoid erogenous zones – at least at first – and to identify areas of your partner's body that he or she did not guess could be so exquisitely erotic. As mentioned, all parts of a woman's body are potential pleasure zones. Neck, ears, back, sides are highly sensitive, yet often sadly neglected by lovers. A man, too, enjoys feeling a woman's delicate touch on his neck or back, perhaps brushing his stomach, chest or shoulders with her fingertips.

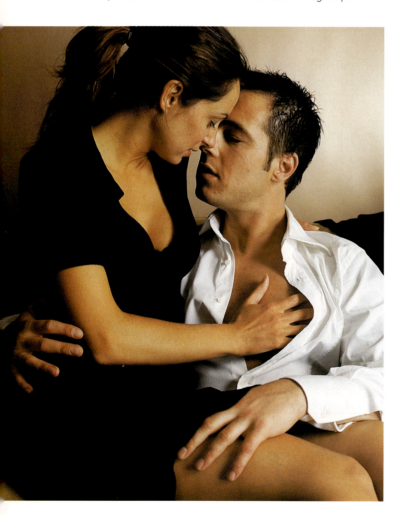

After her confidence has increased still more, he should feel the whole of her body with his hands, and kiss her all over. Some women like to be talked to in the most loving way, others in the most lustful way...

The art for both partners is to keep a light teasing touch. Whenever you are aware of getting a strong response from one part of the body, move on to new areas of arousal. Ask your partner what feels nice and in turn say how and where you enjoy being touched. Don't be afraid to say – tactfully – if some parts of the body are out of bounds at this stage, or if your lover's touch is not quite having the desired effect. You can do this by moving their hands to show them what you'd like. If your partner seems to be becoming too aroused too soon, switch to less sensitive but still potentially arousing regions of the body, slowing movements in order to keep the stimulation going but without bringing your partner to the boil too early.

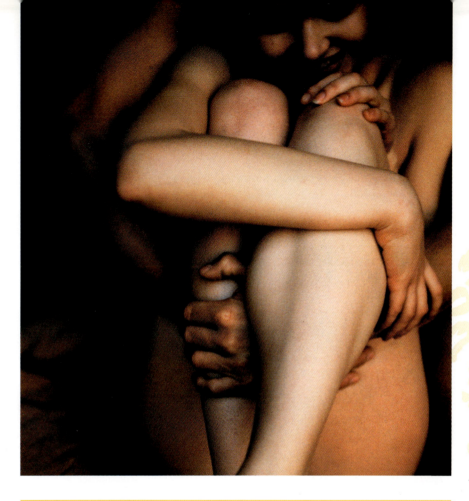

THE
EMBRACE

The Kama Sutra identifies several forms of embrace. They include:

- *The twining of a creeper* Here the man is standing and the woman clings to him as a creeper twines round a tree. She bends his head down to hers with the desire of kissing him, embraces him and looks lovingly towards him.
- *Climbing tree* This time the man is standing and the woman places one of her feet on his foot, and the other on one of his thighs. She passes one of her arms round his back, and the other on his shoulders, as if to climb him for a kiss.
- *Milk and water* In this position the woman sits on her lover's lap. The two embrace as if entering into each other's body.

ABOVE LEFT

Tender touches express your innermost feelings for each other and show that your relationship is fuelled by the power of love as well as lust.

UNDRESSING EACH OTHER

BELOW
Undress each other as deliciously slowly as you can, taking every opportunity to tease and tantalize. Thoroughly explore each area of your lover's body that you expose before uncovering the next part ...

You may decide to retire to the bedroom to continue the fun. Or you might prefer to stay where you are, in the living room, say, and enjoy the delights of curling up on a sofa or lying on the floor together, petting like teenagers. Take your time getting undressed. Slowly peeling to reveal more of your body to your partner adds to the excitement. Unless you are both so highly aroused that you just want to rip each other's clothes off, it's better to take things slowly now, undoing each zip and button with painstaking care, to delay the moment as long as possible. Kiss and stroke each new area of flesh that is uncovered, and remember to pay each other compliments, or simply whisper sexy words of encouragement, so that both partners have little chance to feel self-conscious.

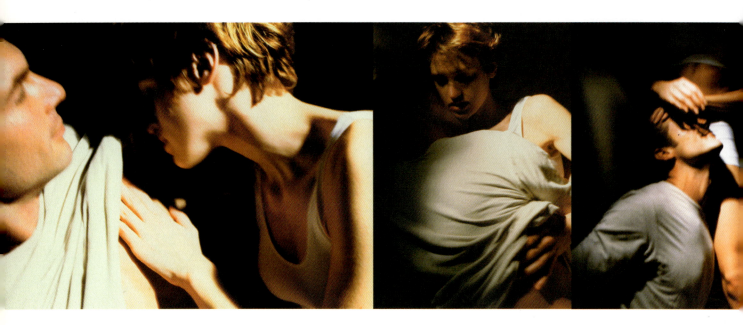

You can prolong the fun by pretending to have difficulty undoing a belt, or unfastening a bra strap and let your hands stray to sensitive zones, as if unintentionally, to inflame your lover even more. If and when you move on to intercourse is up to you. However, you can now prolong the sensual mood by giving each other a sensual massage. This is particularly helpful if you or your partner are still feeling tense, and not yet in the right mood for lovemaking.

UNDRESSING **EACH OTHER** 45

*Some women enjoy themselves with
closed eyes in silence, others make a great noise over it,
and some almost faint away. The great art is to
ascertain what gives them the greatest pleasure, and
what specialities they like best.*

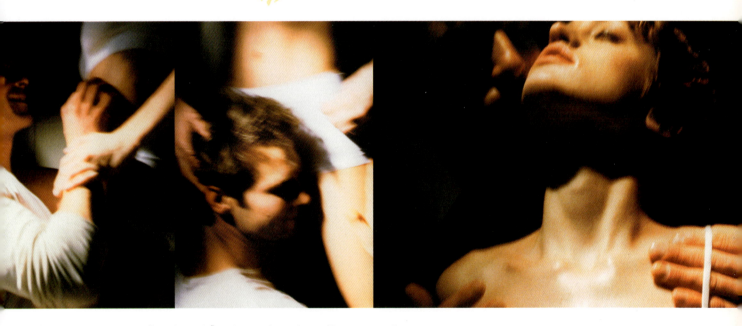

*He should place his hands upon her
thighs and massage them,
and if he succeeds in this he should then
massage the joints of her thighs...*

ABOVE LEFT
... and if you've timed it right, as the last item of clothing falls to the floor your partner will be afire with desire.

SENSUAL MASSAGE

In some parts of India, massage is known as 'shampoo'. This term also refers to head massage, still practised on Indian street corners today, involving soapy lather or oils, and it is where the modern meaning of 'shampoo' originates from. Indian massage can be gentle and relaxing or vigorous and stimulating. It is especially enjoyable as sensual massage, and is recommended in the Kama Sutra as an ideal preliminary to lovemaking, especially when combined with exotic oils and scents.

Partners can take turns to massage each other so that both share the delightful experience. This ensures massage not only becomes a physical experience but also an emotional one promoting caring, sharing and unselfish feelings, as each person concentrates solely on their partner's pleasure. Sensual massage is a way of using touch to heighten the senses and to enhance your awareness of each other. It can aid communication, build up trust and strengthen commitment. Massage also provides yet another opportunity to explore your lover's body to find new areas of sensitivity.

BELOW
For a romantic massage, oil your hands well and try to maintain intimacy by keeping at least one hand in contact with your partner's body at all times.

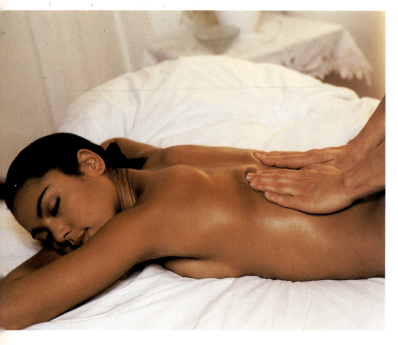

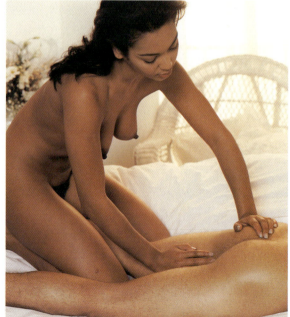

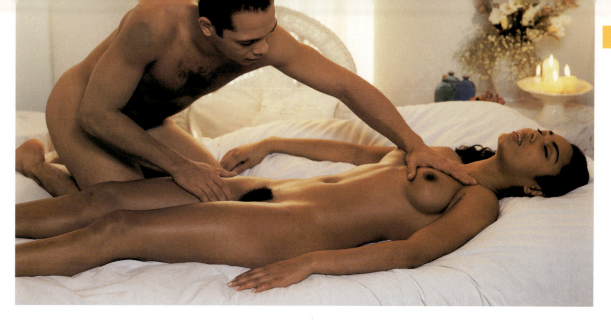

PREPARING FOR MASSAGE

Before you begin a massage, make sure the room is warm, draught-free and as quiet and peaceful as possible. The easiest position to adopt is for the receiver to lie on a soft, thick towel placed on a firm padded surface, such as a futon, hard mattress or thickly carpeted floor. If you are the one giving the massage, it is best to kneel by the side of your partner. Then you can put your whole body behind your massage, which is less tiring than just using arms and hands. A massage can be given without oils, or you can use baby oil or talcum powder instead, but it is more pleasurable for giver and receiver if a good quality 'base' (or 'carrier' oil) is used such as sweet almond, grapeseed, sunflower or olive oil to lubricate the skin. To this can be added a few drops of essential oils (see page 49), for example, ones that have relaxing and sexually arousing properties.

ABOVE

Alter the types of stroke you use as much as possible, applying the softest touches to delicate areas and increasing pressure on fleshy parts of the body.

A woman who is massaging her lover's body, places her face on his thigh (as if she was sleepy) so as to inflame his passion, and kisses his thigh or great toe.

MASSAGE TECHNIQUES

MASSAGE STROKES

There are many types of stroke you can use, depending on the part of the body and the effect you wish to create:

- *Sweeping strokes* For large areas, use firm pressure and sweep both hands out across the skin, letting your hands glide back.
- *Feather strokes* Use light feather strokes for sensitive regions, with each hand working alternately.
- *Circles* Use the palms on large areas, or the fingertips on small areas.
- *Kneading* For fleshy areas or muscles, knead gently between fingers and thumbs.

If using oil, pour a little onto your hands and rub them together to warm it first. Now spread the oil over your partner's body, using light strokes that sweep over the skin, following the contours of the body. Apply more pressure over fleshy parts of the body and use delicate strokes over bony areas. If you notice tense or knotted areas of muscle, most likely in the shoulders, upper arms or lower back, you can relax them by kneading or by pressing with the thumbs, using small circular movements. Be guided by intuition and your partner's responses in locating sensual areas you can devote more attention to, or sensitive regions to avoid. The one giving the massage should enjoy the experience too. So stay relaxed and unhurried and take time to relish the feel of your partner's body.

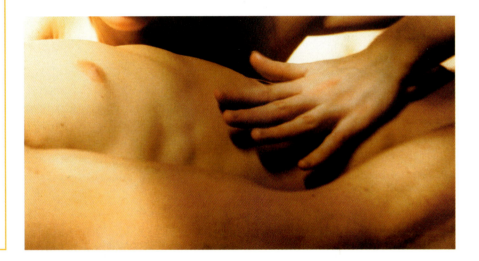

Begin by massaging the back of the body, starting with the neck, arms, shoulders and upper back and slowly moving down to the lower back, buttocks and the backs of the legs to finish with the ankles and feet. Now ask your partner to turn over so you can work on the front of the body, starting with the shoulders and arms and moving down over the chest, abdomen, legs and feet. If this is a purely sensual massage, avoid spending too long on sexually sensitive areas such as breasts, thighs, buttocks and especially genitals. But if this is an erotic massage, your partner will soon be feeling relaxed, contented and in a highly receptive state when you start to stimulate him or her sexually.

ABOVE RIGHT
Reserve featherlight strokes for exquisitely sensitive areas of the body.

MASSAGE TECHNIQUES   49

ESSENTIAL OILS

There are many essential oils to choose from. Each has its own unique therapeutic qualities. The following are good choices for lovers as they have relaxing and aphrodisiac qualities. Use one (or mix up to three) of the following: cedarwood, cinnamon, clary sage, geranium, jasmine, patchouli, rose, rosewood, sandalwood, ylang-ylang in the ratio of 10 to 15 drops of essential oil to five teaspoons of a base oil.

Warning: Essential oils are highly concentrated and must always be diluted by blending with a base oil before applying to the skin. If you are pregnant or suffering from a long-term medical condition, seek expert advice before using essential oils. Avoid massaging over broken or inflamed skin or problem areas such as varicose veins, sores or bruises.

BELOW
Soap and water make an impromptu body lotion – ideal for a spontaneous massage in the shower.

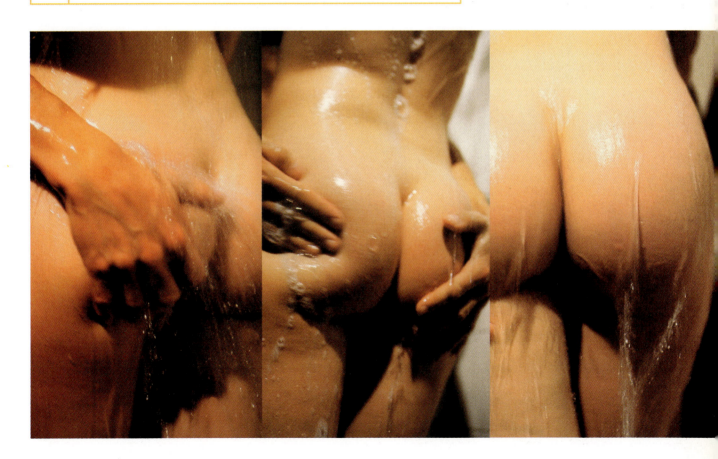

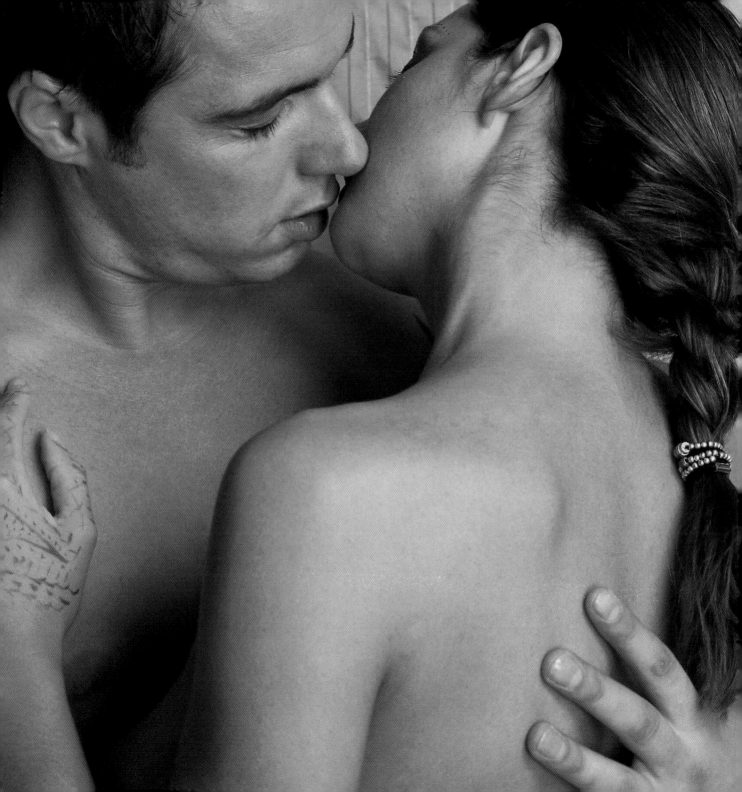

THE SEXUAL ENCOUNTER

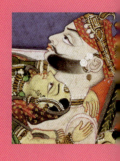

Anything may take place at any time, for love does not care for time or order.

Lovemaking is the ultimate physical expression of a couple's feelings for each other. It usually starts with the kiss, that most intimate of non-genital contacts, and may include tender caresses of petting and foreplay, the erotic charge of manual and oral stimulation, and the divine union of intercourse itself, culminating in blissful climactic release. The Kama Sutra was way ahead of its time in emphasizing mutual pleasure and this is still the most important lesson Vatsyayana offers us today. Sex should be an unselfish act; two lovers delighting in the knowledge that each partner is enjoying the experience as much as the other.

Another lesson from the Kama Sutra is that nothing two consenting adults do together to express their love can be regarded as shameful or reason for guilt. However, it is important, too, that neither partner feels obliged to undertake any sex act they do not enjoy or feel comfortable with or, above all, that puts their health (and life) at risk. With this is mind, never forget the safer sex message (see pages 120–1). If your partner's sexual history is unknown to you, use barrier contraception, or abstain from penetrative sex (after all, there's lots of other fun things you can do together).

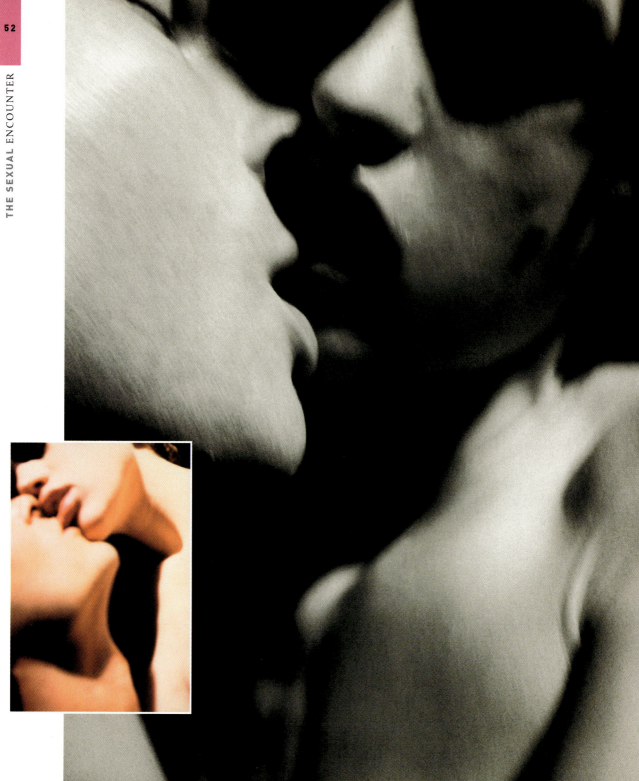

THE KAMA ART OF THE KISS

As a journey of a thousand miles starts with but a single step so the voyage of sexual discovery begins with a simple action – the kiss. The mouth, and especially the lips and tongue, is among the most sensitive parts of the body, covered with nerve endings that relay powerful signals to the brain's limbic system, which regulates emotional responses. Indeed, a larger area of the brain is given over to sensory signals from the mouth than from the genitals. The mouth is supremely versatile, capable of passionate pressure or a gossamer touch guaranteed to inflame a lover – little wonder that the Kama Sutra devotes much space to the art of kissing. A kiss expresses so much – attraction, love, arousal and desire; the first kiss marks the change in a couple's relationship from friendship to intimacy. It strengthens that all-important emotional bond. So never miss an opportunity to exchange kisses, and not only when you meet and part, or as a prelude to sex. For example, if one partner is occupied, perhaps reading or preparing a meal, a tender kiss on the cheek or under the ear expresses so much.

KISSING TECHNIQUES

If your kisses start light and delicate, there is scope to increase the pressure slowly, allowing the passion to build. Lick your lips and then plant small kisses over your lover's mouth and cheeks. And don't neglect the jaw-line, the nape of the neck or the ears, which are particularly sensitive. Trace a line of kisses from one ear to the other, lightly following the curve of your lover's throat. Press your partner's lower lip between your own and suck, applying a light vacuum pressure. Then flick it gently with your tongue. As your desire mounts, the kiss will become stronger as you press your lips firmly against each other.

Begin to probe your partner's mouth with your tongue, delighting in the intimacy of the moment – the Kama Sutra describes this as 'fighting of the tongues', each one pressing against the other, and then tracing the contours of your partner's mouth (see Kama Kissing, page 54). In Vatsyayana's day, entering your lover's mouth with the tongue symbolized the act of sexual penetration to follow. As the kissing grows more passionate, it easily and naturally leads to greater sexual intimacy. But no matter how powerful your feelings now, try not to rush this stage. Kissing, more than any other romantic

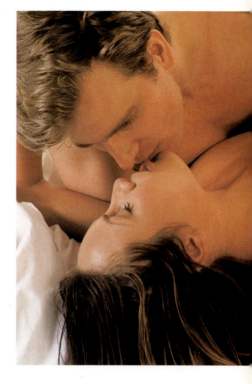

ABOVE
More than a mere entrée to romance, kissing is a powerful 'congress of the lips' that triggers arousal and heightens passion.

FAR LEFT
The kiss of the upper lip, as described in the Kama Sutra, expresses tenderness and focuses all your senses on your lover.

activity, reveals the emotional depth of the feelings two people have for each other. Any delay now makes the lovemaking to come even more intense.

By moistening your lips with your tongue again, you can trace wet kisses around, for example, your lover's neck, and then gently blow on the glistening marks you've left to make the skin tingle. From the neck you can plant kisses on all exposed areas of skin – chest, cleavage, shoulders, arms … there is no limit. All parts of the body respond to the soft caress of the mouth, especially the nipples and inner thigh, so the art of kissing in all its forms is a skill that should not be underestimated.

Kissing is of four kinds: moderate, contracted, pressed and soft, according to the different parts of the body which are kissed.

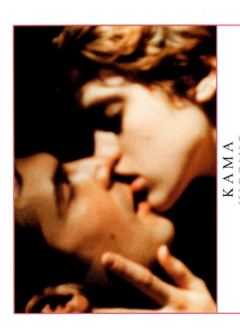

KAMA KISSING

Vatsyayana describes a dozen or more forms of kissing, including:

- *The nominal kiss* Lightly touching the mouth of your lover with your own.
- *The throbbing kiss* Touching the lip that is pressed into your mouth by only moving the lower lip, not the upper one.
- *The touching kiss* Touching your lover's lip with your tongue.
- *The straight kiss* Bringing the lips of the two lovers into direct contact with each other.
- *The pressed kiss* Pressing the lower lip with much force.
- *The greatly pressed kiss* Taking hold of your lover's lower lip with two fingers and after touching it with the tongue, pressing it with great force with your lip.
- *The kiss of the upper lip* Pressing your lips against your partner's upper lip, while he or she kisses your lower lip.
- *The clasping kiss* Taking your lover's two lips between your own.
- *Fighting of the tongues* With your tongue, touching the tongue, teeth and palate of your lover.

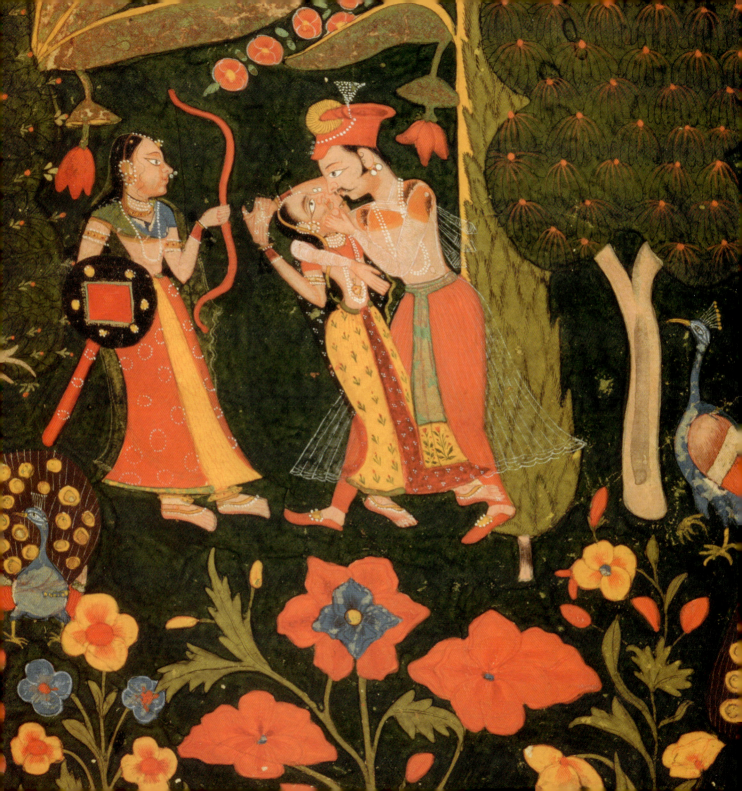

PETTING AND FOREPLAY

FAR RIGHT
By word or gesture, use positive encouragement to let your lover know you like what they're doing.

BELOW
Vatsyayana stresses the sexual caress, which allows time for passion to grow.

If you have already taken time to explore your partner's sensual body, you'll have a good idea how and where your partner likes to be touched. If not, now is the time to find out. As well as needing a long build-up, a woman is capable of multiple orgasms, so a man can never give his partner too much erotic stimulation at this stage. As ever, the Kama Sutra's message is to start slowly and gently, taking every opportunity to tease and play, and slowly increasing the intensity as you feel your partner's passion grow. A man usually becomes more quickly aroused than a woman so she should take care not to stimulate her partner too much too soon. When he has climaxed once, however, and is ready to resume lovemaking, she can use more intense stimulation to rekindle his passion, with less risk he will climax prematurely.

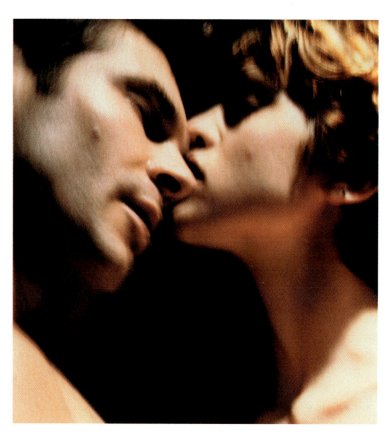

Aim to build up anticipation by avoiding the most sexually sensitive areas at first. An imaginative lover can find ways to tantalize a partner, by slowly approaching erogenous zones and then moving away again, never quite reaching the magic spot, leaving the lover begging for more. For a woman, lower back, shoulders, and backs of the knees are areas of potential sensual pleasure that are often ignored. Her partner can then stimulate the more highly charged areas, such as the abdomen, buttocks and inner thighs, starting with a gentle touch and increasing the pressure as his partner slowly begins to respond. He can use his fingers to stroke, rub and gently squeeze softer regions of his lover's body while tenderly licking and sucking more delicately sensitive areas.

Most women enjoy having their breasts stroked and squeezed, and their nipples sucked. But some women say men don't know how hard to squeeze their breasts, and are either too firm, or not firm enough. So let your partner show you how much pressure she likes. For some women, having their breasts expertly fondled by a sensitive lover is an intensely arousing sensation that can even bring them close to climax. Other women say their breasts are not very sensitive, and prefer a partner to focus on areas such as thighs, abdomen, bottom and perineum. Explore and you'll find the magic buttons.

Men relish a woman's teasing caress – hand, mouth or both – on their chest, back, legs and buttocks. A man's feet are especially sensitive, and he may find having his toes sucked an unexpected delight. This is one way a woman's imagination can enhance her partner's pleasure. Her hands may find areas of arousal in unforeseen places.

After gaining this point he should touch her private parts, should loosen her girdle and the knot of her dress, and turning up her lower garment should stroke the joints of her naked thighs.

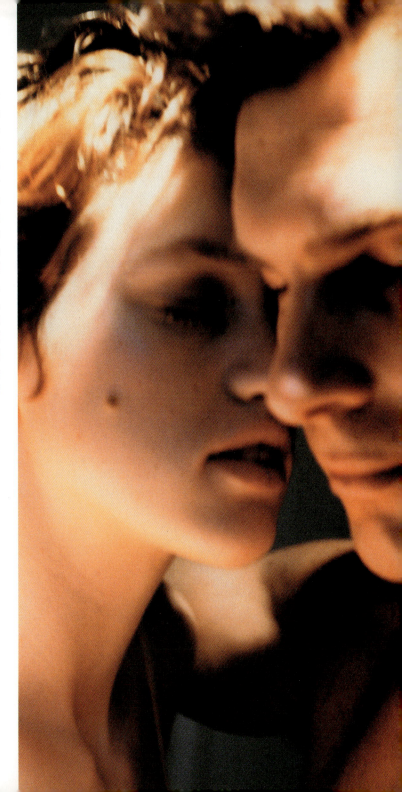

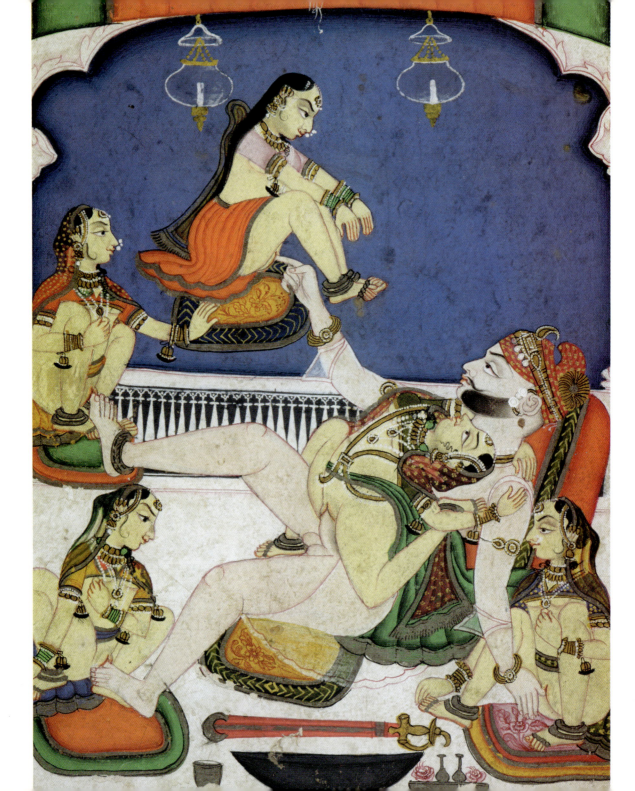

Response is important: Guide your partner's hand to your own unique target zones. If your lover does anything that feels particularly good, let him or her know. But don't assume you'll be told when you've hit the spot. The powerful sensations your lover is experiencing now may have left him or her speechless. In that case, you can assume you are getting it right! Be aware of the groans, gasps of pleasure, deep breathing and other sounds your partner makes, and the movements of the body. For example, if a woman pushes against your hand it's a sure sign you've found the right place and she wants more of the same, possibly with more pressure.

He should rub her yoni with his hands or fingers and not begin to have intercourse with her until she becomes excited or experiences pleasure.

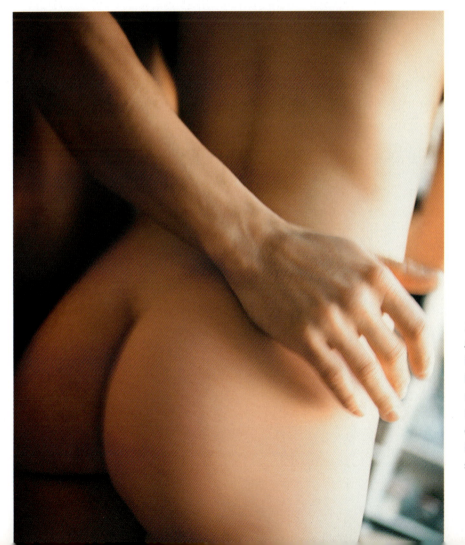

LEFT
A woman may show she is becoming aroused by little more than slight body movements, a tensing of muscles and the softest of gasps, but an attentive lover looks out for these subtle signs.

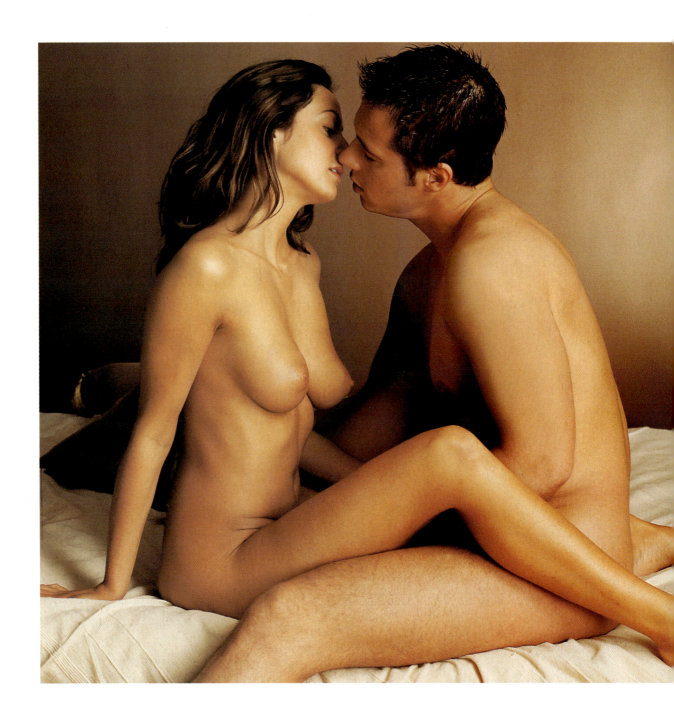

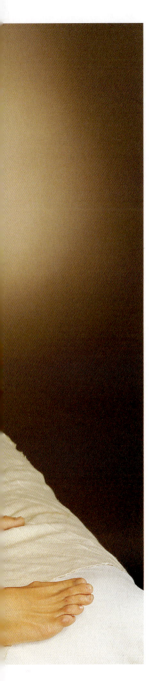

MUTUAL MASTURBATION

Having delighted in all the other erogenous areas, it's now time to concentrate on the principal pleasure zones. A woman may worry about handling a man's penis and testicles too roughly, concerned about hurting him. Men, however, often say their partners don't apply enough pressure. One way to teach a lover is to guide his or her hand, increasing or reducing pressure and friction as necessary. Or watch as a partner pleasures him or herself. Treat it as a private peep show, and enjoy the sight of your lover caressing his or her body, while they take pleasure in the effect this is having on you. If you want to, you can take over and bring your partner to climax or switch to another form of lovemaking, such as oral sex (see pages 64–75).

TOUCH AND LEARN

Sex therapists believe the ability to respond sexually is not innate and has to be learned first. In the absence of an experienced sexual partner who can show you what your body is capable of, this knowledge usually comes through masturbation. Studies show that women who learn about their own sexual nature through self-pleasuring are more likely to have good sexual relationships with partners. In this way, they discover where and how they like to be stimulated, and can relay this store of knowledge to a lover.

When you masturbate, don't limit your touch to your breasts and sex organs but include other areas of the body that can generate arousing sensations. You can also use this moment to develop the power of your imagination and visualize an erotic scene. Combine tactile feelings with a secret fantasy, such as being made love to in the woods, on a beach, in a car or in public, that you can use to heighten your arousal when you are with a partner. (For more on fantasy, see page 99.)

FAR LEFT

Mutual pleasuring, accompanied by gentle kisses and whispered words of tenderness, is both intimate and powerfully arousing.

BREAKING THE PATTERN

Fact: Men are less inhibited about self-pleasure than women (sexologist Alfred Kinsey said 98 per cent of men owned up to masturbation, and the other 2 per cent lied!). But men must learn how to regulate their sexual responses. During puberty, when males masturbate for the first time, they can get into the habit of reaching their climax too rapidly (perhaps through fear of discovery). Later, this may develop into an ingrained pattern of hurried lovemaking when they are with a sexual partner, even leading to premature ejaculation. Making sex a total sensual experience – as extolled in the Kama Sutra – helps a man to break this pattern, or not develop it in the first place.

HAND STIMULATION – FOR WOMEN

BELOW

The best way to show how you want to be touched is to let a lover watch while you pleasure yourself.

BELOW RIGHT

The subtlety of a woman's touch can show a man what his body is really capable of and stimulating him this way can be highly arousing for her too.

When masturbating a woman, keep in mind the theme running through this book that a slow, steady build-up is more arousing than too much stimulation too soon. Notice your partner's responses so you know what she likes. And don't be surprised if she brings your hand back to an area where she particularly enjoys being touched. You could start with long light strokes along the soft skin of the inner thigh, approaching but not quite reaching, the vulva. Now use slightly firmer, circular movements over the pubic mound, getting tantalizingly closer to – but without touching – the clitoral area.

As you feel your partner's passion build, turn your attention to her vulva. With your index and middle finger in a V-shape, very gently rub along the outer labia, slowly at first, then increase the friction. Moisten a finger and rub it along the edges of her labia and then squeeze one labium gently between finger and thumb. Don't be in too much of a hurry to leave an area you are stimulating (and take time to relish the feel of her). If you are getting little response, move on. But if you think she is ready for more intense stimulation, rub the clitoral area with your palm, using steadily increasing pressure. If your partner can stand the intensity of the feeling, rubbing a well-lubricated thumb and forefinger either side of her clitoris will drive her wild. Otherwise, rub the clitoral hood.

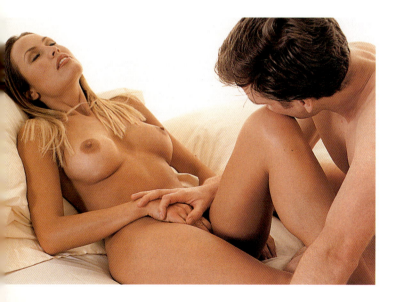

Once your lover is fully aroused and her vagina well lubricated, you can gently insert your middle finger (usually the longest one), rubbing the vaginal entrance and then stroking the front wall over the G-spot. You may need to use a little artificial lubricant (see page 78) if your partner is not quite moist enough. At the same time, rub the clitoral area with your palm if your hand is at the right angle to do so. As she begins to climax, you'll notice her muscles tense and you may feel her vagina throb as it contracts rhythmically. She may cry out, but don't expect her to. You'll soon learn her unique pattern of orgasmic responses. Maintain the same pace and pressure until she relaxes, when you'll know her orgasm has passed. This may take 20–30 seconds, or sometimes even longer.

HAND STIMULATION – FOR MEN

When masturbating a man, a slow build-up is just as important as it is for a woman, but for a different reason. A man can find being masturbated by his partner such a powerful stimulus that he climaxes too soon. So your aim should be to prolong his pleasure for as long as possible. Start with long, slow stroking movements along his inner thigh or lower abdomen, or perhaps gently tug at the pubic hairs. Lightly cup his testicles in your hand and gently squeeze and then release. If he enjoys this, you could repeat it a few times.

Now encircle the shaft of his penis with your thumb and forefinger and slowly rub it up and down. Pause occasionally to stroke the frenulum, or squeeze the foreskin, if he is uncircumcised, and then roll it back and lightly stroke the glans itself. Rubbing the head of the penis is often more pleasurable if you use generous amounts of lubricant first, especially if your partner is circumcised.

If men and women act according to each other's liking, their love for each other will not be lessened even in one hundred years.

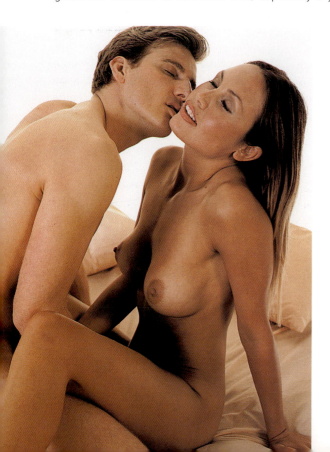

Some men may find that, without lubrication, the glans is too sensitive to stimulate directly. As you stroke the shaft of the penis, steadily increase your hand speed and pressure until your partner indicates that the stimulus is just right. Or let your partner guide your hand to show you how he likes it. Rubbing closer to the glans gives more intense stimulus. If he starts to climax too soon, stop and let his erection soften slightly and then start again. Slow the pace as he begins to ejaculate but don't stop until he relaxes, when you'll know his climax has passed.

GOOD VIBRATIONS

A vibrator or other sexual aid can help men and women explore the depth of their own sexual responses and their partners'. Focus on small areas of the body, or sweep over larger areas of flesh, delivering a more intense sensation than can be achieved by hand alone (see also Sex Toys, pages 109–10).

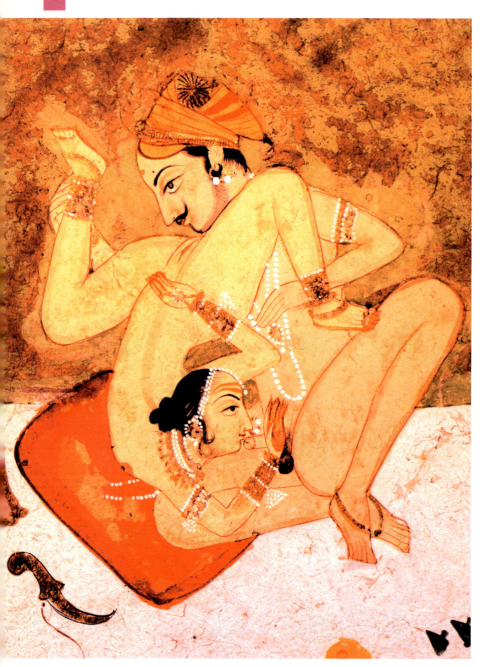

ORAL SEX AND POSITIONS

Sensual, erotic, emotionally highly charged – and with the added thrill of knowing you're doing something some would regard as taboo – oral sex seems like the ultimate sexual experience. It is certainly the most intimate form of lovemaking, and takes any sexual relationship to a different plane. But it also involves a high degree of trust on the part of both partners. For a woman, giving and receiving oral sex requires patience and sensitivity if she is to relax and enjoy the experience to the full. In the Kama Sutra, oral sex is called *auparishtaka* or 'mouth congress' and the various forms are given such inventive names as 'biting the sides', 'swallowing up' and 'sucking a mango'.

When performed on a woman, oral sex is called 'cunnilingus'. A woman can find this form of sex powerfully exciting because of the intimacy, the range of sensations it can produce and the knowledge she is doing something 'extraordinary'. Once a woman's thighs are spread well apart, a man's mouth can reach and explore all parts of her vulva, especially the inner labia and clitoris, and then push his tongue into the warm recesses of her vagina. To avoid causing discomfort, it is a good idea to cover the teeth with the lips and gently press the tender flesh with the lips and mouth. Oral sex is more pleasant for a woman if her partner is clean-shaven, as a bristly face on the sensitive skin of the thigh can cause irritation and even a painful rash.

If her partner uses care and sensitivity, a woman should have no difficulty climaxing with oral sex. Many experience multiple orgasms for the first time this way. Men also enjoy giving oral sex and can be powerfully aroused by the sight, scent, taste and intense emotional sensations experienced by such close, intimate contact with a woman.

POSITIONS FOR CUNNILINGUS

Any position that brings a man's face in close proximity to his partner's vulva is fine for cunnilingus. Just make sure you get comfortable at the beginning so you can sustain the pose until your lover has climaxed. Nothing spoils the mood like an attack of cramp just as your partner is going into orbit. The simplest position is for your partner to lie on her back on a bed with her feet on the floor and her legs spread comfortably wide. You can kneel on the floor in front of her with your face between her thighs. In this position, you have good control over your movements and can tease your partner as you choose. You are well placed to reach forward and feel her breasts, or stroke her abdomen and thighs.

There are many variations on this theme. For example, the woman can sit in a chair, with one leg slung over an arm of the chair or over your shoulder, resting her foot on your back. This position is great for spontaneous moments of lovemaking in the living room (even in the office) as she can remain fully clothed, only needing to lift her skirt up to her thighs. She doesn't even need to remove her underwear, as you can apply your mouth through her panties – a great experience for both of you.

Alternatively, you can lie on your back and your partner can kneel with her thighs placed either side of your head, and slowly lower her groin onto your face. This position gives her total control, as you are virtually trapped and she can place her body exactly where she wants you to stimulate her. She can even lift herself away from you to slow the pace. The sense of empowerment that this position offers can be highly arousing for her. From where you are lying (assuming she's left your arms free), you can use your hands to stroke the curves of her back and buttocks.

Some women of the harem, when they are amorous, do the acts of the mouth on the yonis of one another, and men do the same thing with women. The way of doing this should be known from kissing the mouth.

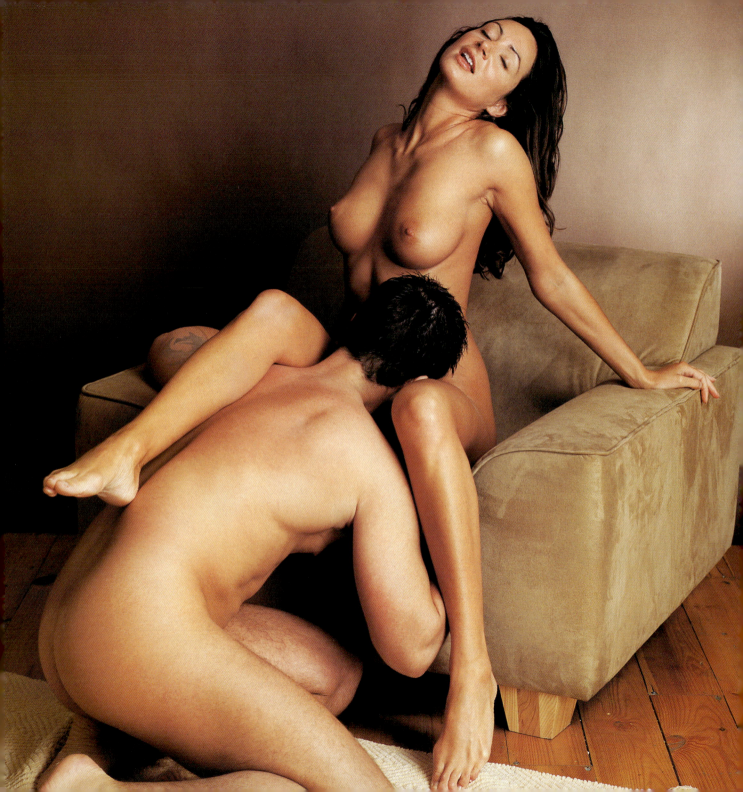

CUNNILINGUS TECHNIQUES

As with manual stimulation, aim to let your partner's sexual tension build slowly. Her arousal will be greatly enhanced if you spend time caressing her entire body before giving oral sex. Start by caressing her breasts, perhaps licking and sucking her nipples, before slowly working down her abdomen. Take your time before reaching her pubic mound – she knows where you're heading so the suspense just adds to her pleasure. Use delicate teasing movements of your lips and tongue, and increase the stimulation as her passion mounts. Her responses should indicate whether she likes what you are doing. Once your face is between her legs, you can nibble her inner thigh gently with your lips and run your tongue over the soft skin of her perineum – easier to reach from this angle. Next, caress the skin between thigh and vulva, first one side and then the other. Pause for effect, gently parting her pubic hair and take time to enjoy the sight of her. Run your tongue upwards along the vulva in one long, firm but gentle stroke. This sends a shock wave of pleasure through her body. She may even give a little gasp of surprise.

Vary your movements and the regions being stimulated, perhaps alternating between kissing the pubic mound and running your tongue along the moist lining of the labia, or using delicate tongue flicks to make her clitoris tingle. Now you can increase the stimulation, perhaps stroking one part with your fingertips while your mouth teases another area of the body, or running your hands over her breasts or thighs. Even the tip of your nose can be brought in to play, nuzzling her clitoris while you tongue the vaginal opening. Once you feel she is ready to climax, push your tongue deep into her vagina, relishing the love juices that should be flowing freely now. At the same time, rub your fingers over her clitoral hood, or along her thighs and buttocks. Continue the stimulation until she relaxes and you know her climax has passed.

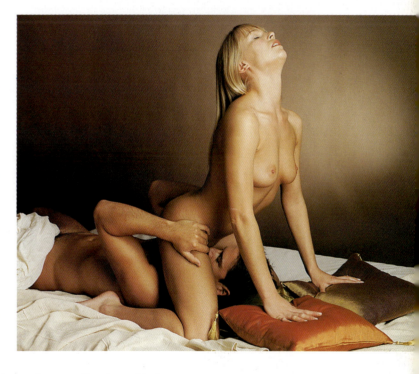

FAR LEFT
Reclining in a soft armchair, while her lover pays her intimate lip service, a woman can abandon herself utterly to amazing sensations.

ABOVE
Straddling her man, while he lies below her with his face between her thighs, can give a woman a strong feeling of power.

THE SEXUAL ENCOUNTER

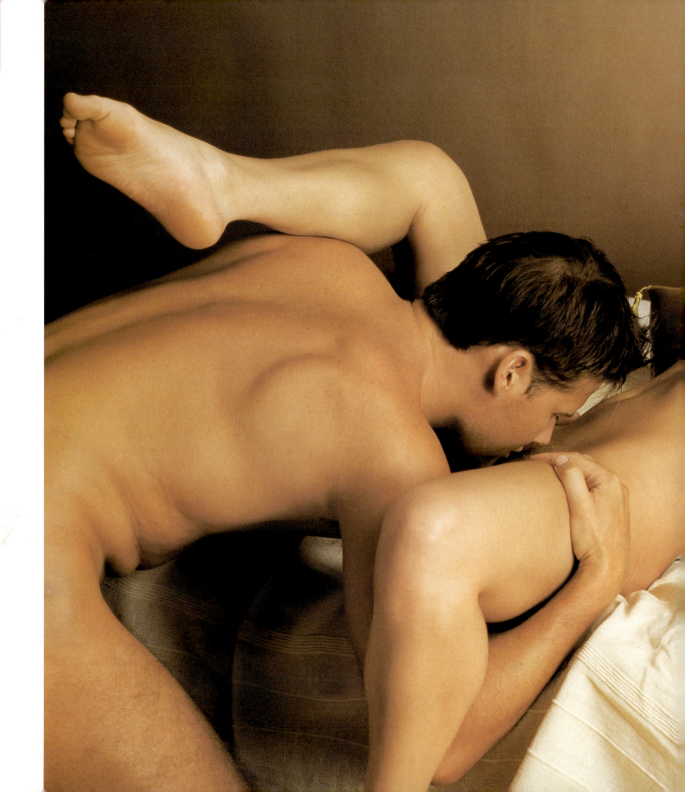

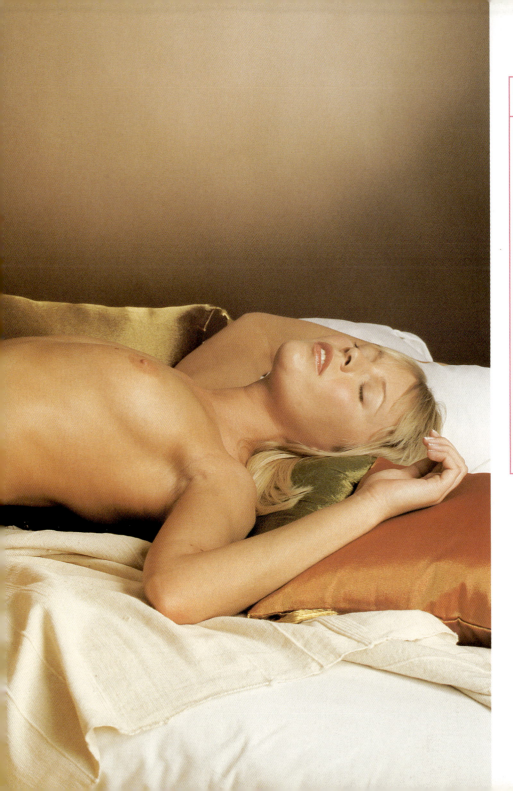

SEX TIP

To become expert at performing oral sex on a woman it can help to strengthen the tongue muscles. Give your tongue a regular workout by stretching it out as far as it will go and circling it round and round. Now try to touch your nose with it and then reach down towards your chin. A great way to strengthen the tongue is to lick out a small container of yogurt, pushing the tip into the corners. Develop this skill and you'll be an instant hit with your lover.

LEFT

Lying at the edge of the bed is a blissfully relaxing position for a woman, and it is easy for her partner to reach her most deliciously sensitive areas with his lips and tongue.

RIGHT
Sitting in a chair for oral sex, a man can guide his partner's head with his hand, but he must take care not to restrict her freedom of movement.

FAR RIGHT
Many men feel that oral sex is one of the greatest sexual gifts a woman can give, as she 'worships' his body with her mouth.

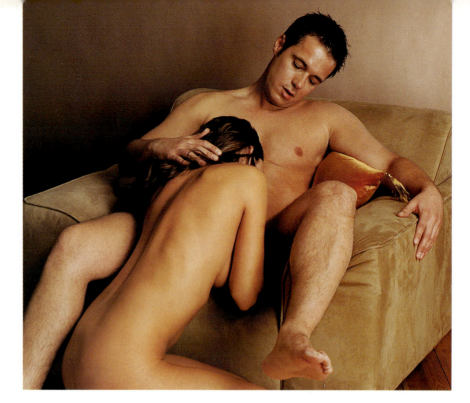

These things being done secretly … how can it be known what any person will do at any particular time, and for any particular purpose?

POSITIONS FOR FELLATIO

Oral sex performed on males is called 'fellatio'. For many men, the delights of having a warm, moist, flexible mouth and tongue paying lip service to the sex organs are beyond compare. His partner can control the frequency and form of stimulation, and so increase his pleasure. There are several positions for fellatio. The man can sit in a chair while his partner kneels between his thighs, or approaches him from the side. Alternatively, he can stand while his partner kneels in front of him, with her hands on his buttocks or the backs of his thighs for support. The woman has most control if her partner lies on his back and she leans over and takes him into her mouth. From this position she can easily move her head to kiss, lick and caress the penis from all angles, and can also stroke the shaft. Another position is for the woman to lie on her back while her partner straddles her chest, leaning over her and taking his weight on hands and knees. However, this position is suitable for very close, trusting relationships only, as a man is in a powerful position and his partner has little freedom of movement. Before agreeing to this, she must feel confident he will avoid thrusting too deeply and will withdraw when she asks.

TECHNIQUES FOR FELLATIO

Fellatio is so arousing that your partner may find it impossible to stop himself ejaculating, so aim to regulate the pace and pressure of the stimulation you give, to delay ejaculation as long as possible. Be aware of his responses, such as a tightening in the muscles of legs, abdomen and buttocks, that show he is close to orgasm. You may then slow the pace, or let his erection decline before continuing again. Oral sex can be reserved for times when a man has climaxed once and wants to be re-aroused.

Start by kissing and lightly stroking non-genital areas, such as the chest, lower abdomen or thighs, before slowly working towards his genitals. Your partner might enjoy you paying special regard to the delicate skin of the scrotum, using your lips or tongue, or squeezing the testicles gently while you turn your attention to his penis. You can hold the shaft of the penis while you lightly kiss and lick the glans. Or stroke his thighs while you stimulate him with your mouth alone. Perhaps use your lips on the shaft, sucking or licking upwards as you work your way towards the glans itself. Now swirl your tongue over the glans or take it into your mouth, sucking it gently.

It is, of course, your choice how much of the penis you take into your mouth. At this stage your partner can control your movements by placing his hands on your head, but you must be able to withdraw. He should tell you when he is close to climaxing so you can decide whether you want to let him ejaculate in your mouth. Semen can be safely swallowed, but you might prefer to spit it out into a tissue. Alternatively, you can take his penis from your mouth and bring him to climax with your hand or another part of your body (such as between your breasts).

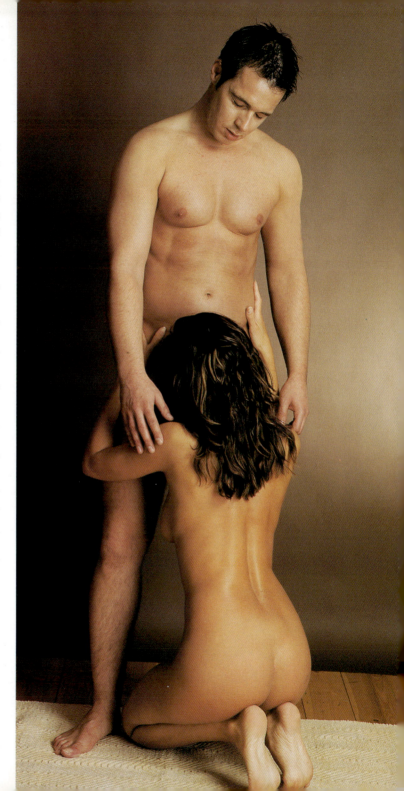

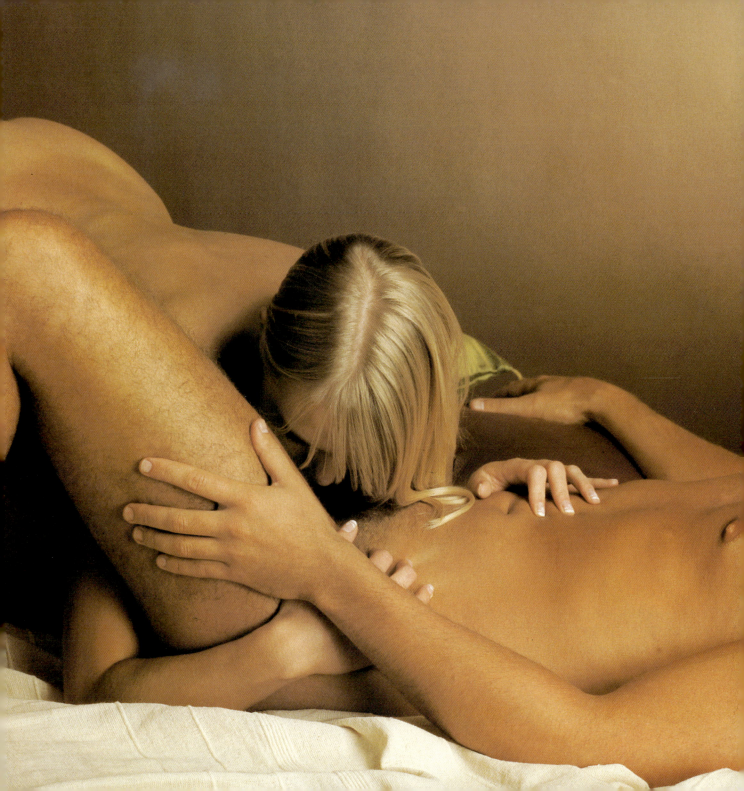

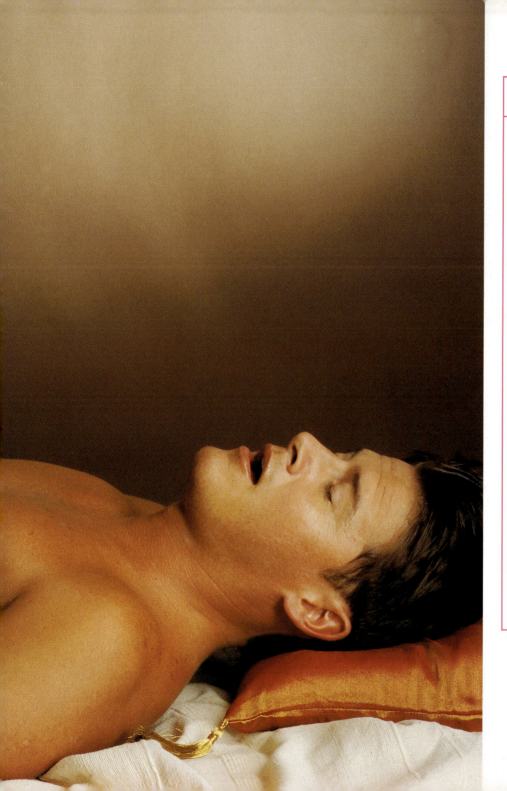

KAMA MOUTH CONGRESS

The Kama Sutra describes fellatio:

- *Nominal congress* The *lingam* is held in the hand, placed between lips and moved about the mouth.
- *Biting the sides* Covering the end of the *lingam* with fingers together like a bud of a flower, the sides are pressed with the lips. The teeth are also used.
- *Outside pressing* The end of the *lingam* is pressed with lips closed together and kissed.
- *Inside pressing* The *lingam* is placed further into the mouth, pressed with the lips and then taken out.
- *Kissing* The *lingam* is held in the hand and kissed as if kissing his lower lip.
- *Rubbing* After kissing, the *lingam* is touched everywhere with the tongue, and the tongue is passed over the end of it.
- *Sucking a mango fruit* Half the *lingam* is put into the mouth, and kissed and sucked with force.
- *Swallowing up* The whole *lingam* is placed in the mouth and pressed to the very end, as if being swallowed up.

LEFT
Fellatio performed lying down allows her to move into the best position.

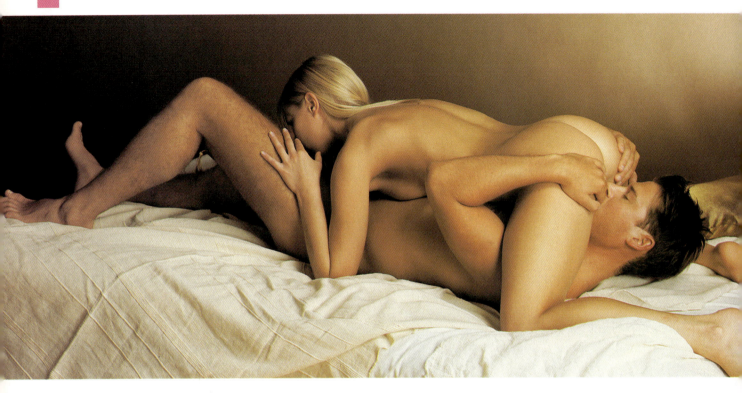

ABOVE
Naughty but nice ... by taking the on-top position, a woman can comfortably pleasure her partner, while enjoying arousing oral stimulation from him.

MUTUAL ORAL SEX

Men and women can use their mouths to pleasure each other simultaneously. The Kama Sutra calls this 'the congress of the crow', but it is better known today as *soixante-neuf* (French for 'sixty-nine'). The name describes the inverted position adopted by couples. If you want to try this, you'll need to find a position that is comfortable for both of you, either on the bed or lying on folded blankets or sheets, or even rugs on the floor. It is easier and safer for the woman if her partner lies on his back and she lies on top with his face between her thighs and her head over his penis. Many couples find it more relaxing to lie on their sides, resting the head on their partner's lower leg.

Soixante-neuf offers a novel and exciting form of sexual stimulus, but there are potential difficulties that may require patience and practise to overcome. For example, it is difficult to concentrate on giving tender oral stimulation when your own body is being racked by earth-shaking sensations caused by your partner's

MUTUAL ORAL SEX   75

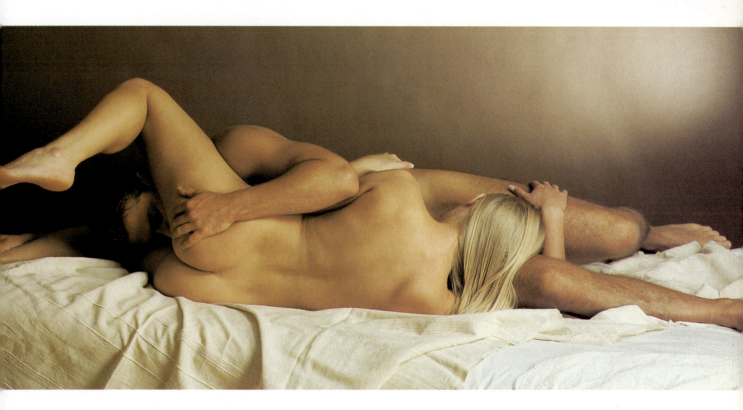

ABOVE
Leisurely loving ... lying on their sides, using their partner's lower thigh as a comfy pillow, a couple can delight in relaxed, unhurried oral sex.

loving attention. There is even a risk one partner may get so excited he – or especially she – bites the other's genitals at the height of passion. Also, oral sex is so arousing for a man he may well climax before his partner is fully sexually satisfied. For all these reasons, it is often best if the man stimulates his partner first, ensuring she is close to climaxing before she turns her attention to him. Alternatively, they could take turns to pleasure each other. Couples may prefer to enjoy mutual oral sex briefly and without continuing right up to orgasm, simply to heighten their arousal, before switching to another sexual position.

> *When a man and woman lie down in an inverted order, with the head of one towards the feet of the other, it is called 'the congress of the crow'.*

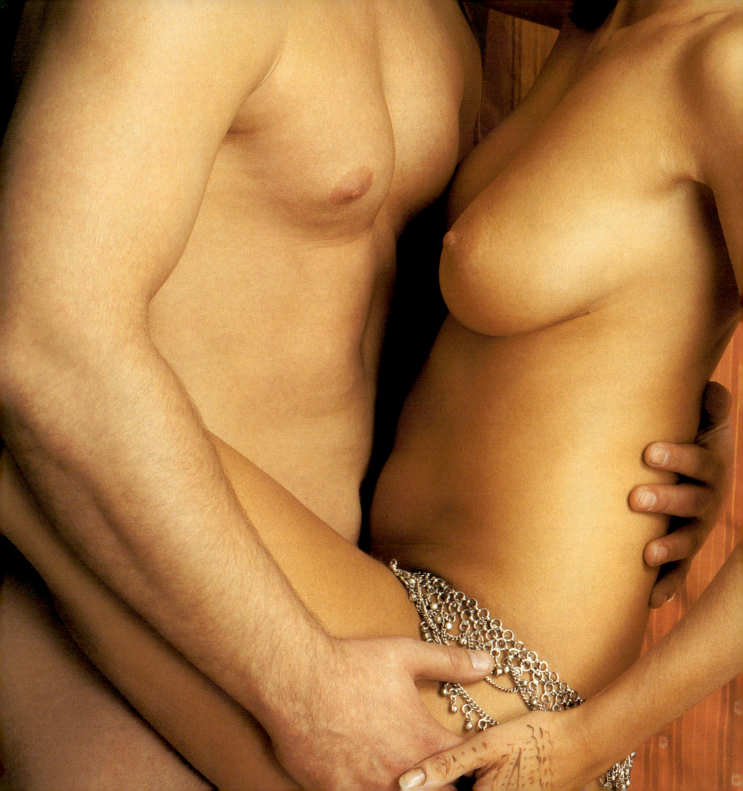

SEXUAL POSITIONS

The congress that takes place between two persons who are attached to one another, and which is done according to their own liking, is called 'spontaneous congress'.

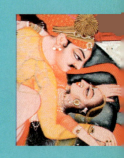

For many lovers, penetrative sex is the only form of intercourse that truly expresses the depth of their feelings for one another. Vatsyayana, who famously said that sex is only sinful if done badly, believed lovers should play an equal part in lovemaking and enjoy equal pleasure. The Kama Sutra is, perhaps, best known for the various sexual positions it describes. Many demonstrate Vatsyayana's philosophy by, for example, limiting a man's range of movement. This slows his rate of thrusting and reduces the stimulation he receives, thereby prolonging intercourse long enough to ensure his partner is satisfied.

Some positions change the angle of penetration, so that the head of the penis stimulates different regions of the vagina, creating new and exciting sensations for both partners. To become fully aroused and to climax, the lovers must move their bodies in harmony. Adopting a more relaxed approach enhances feelings of intimacy, reduces performance pressure and helps strengthen emotional bonds while still ensuring couples enjoy sex to the full.

The Kama Sutra encourages a fluid approach to lovemaking, moving seamlessly from one position to another, exploring the full range of sensation and stimulation two lovers can enjoy. When couples are sexually in tune, their movements synchronize like dancers, each partner knowing instinctively when to adopt a new position or accelerate or slow the pace. This level of understanding comes only with time and practise. But sometimes it just works – the chemistry's right. Many positions described in the Kama Sutra make full use of the body's amazing flexibility. But unless you are confident that you and your partner have the suppleness required, it is best to avoid any position that might lead to muscle, joint or spinal injury, especially if you have a back or joint disorder.

MAN ON TOP

LOVE LUBRICANTS

It is important that a woman is aroused and moist to facilitate comfortable intercourse for both parties. In some cases – especially during extended lovemaking – her natural lubrication may not be enough. In that case it is best to use a proprietary lubricating gel. Use water-based lubricants if you are using rubber (latex) condoms, which can be damaged by petroleum-based types. Plastic (polyurethane) condoms are not damaged by petroleum gels.

There are many positions that allow the man to adopt the dominant on-top position. Best known and most widely practised is the 'missionary position', in which the woman lies on her back with legs parted. The man lies between her thighs and supports his weight on hands or elbows and legs. He then inserts his penis into her vagina and uses rhythmic thrusting movements of his pelvis to create the stimulation he and his partner need to climax. The man can easily control the speed, depth and angle of penetration and his partner can press her feet and legs against the bed to adjust her position slightly to readjust the angle of entry and to aid his actions if she chooses.

This position has advantages and disadvantages. Being face to face, the couple can maintain eye contact and can see and enjoy each other's highly aroused expressions. They can also kiss

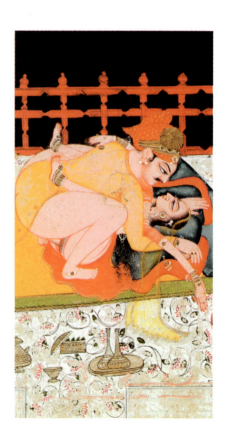

MAN ON TOP

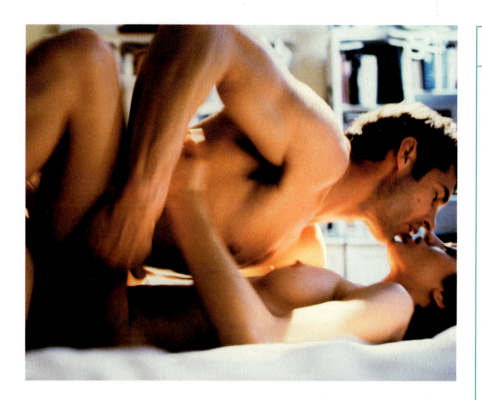

KAMA SEX STROKES

As well as positions, Vatsyayana describes the various strokes a man might use during penetration:

- **Moving the organ forward** The organs are brought together properly and directly.
- **Churning** The *lingam* is held with the hand, and turned all around in the *yoni*.
- **Piercing** The *yoni* is lowered and the upper part of it is struck with the *lingam*.
- **Rubbing** The same thing is done on the lower part of the *yoni*.
- **Pressing** The *yoni* is pressed by the *lingam* for a long time.
- **Giving a blow** The lingam is removed to a distance from the *yoni*, and then forcibly strikes it.
- **Blow of a boar** When only one part of the *yoni* is rubbed.
- **Blow of a bull** When both sides of the *yoni* are rubbed.
- **Sporting of a sparrow** The *lingam* is in the *yoni* and moved up and down frequently, without being taken out. This takes place at the end of intercourse.

tenderly or passionately to maintain that all-important bond. The woman's hands are free to caress her partner's chest, back and buttocks and to reach down to stimulate her labia and clitoris. By keeping an arm free, her partner can caress her body, especially breasts and thighs, and so help her climax. However, this is a passive position for the woman as her freedom to move is restricted, especially if her partner's weight is pressing down on her.

When the lingam is in the yoni, and moved up and down frequently, and without being taken out, it is called the 'sporting of the sparrow'. This takes place at the end of congress.

ABOVE LEFT
Here the man has control over penetration; his partner can tilt her pelvis up in time with his thrusts.

MAN-ON-TOP VARIATIONS

Variations on the 'missionary' theme allow a woman to take a more active part in sex. For example, by placing her feet flat on the bed, she can push up with more force to meet her lover's downward thrusts. Alternatively, by wrapping her legs around his legs, buttocks or waist, she can control his movements and direct his penis to where it gives her most pleasure. If the woman keeps one leg straight and the other wrapped around her partner's waist, she has even more control and can angle herself so that her vulva gets extra stimulation from her partner's thigh. She can easily reach down to caress her pubic mound and clitoral hood in this position.

By supporting himself on his knees and lifting his partner's legs higher, the man can increase the depth of penetration, if they both choose, and align his penis to stimulate different regions of her vagina. If the woman is very flexible, she can place her legs on her partner's shoulders or around his neck. The Kama Sutra calls this the 'yawning position'. Alternatively, she can raise her knees and, keeping her knees and legs together, place her feet against his chest. Vatsyayana

BELOW LEFT
The 'pressed position' is one of the best-known from the Kama Sutra: by tightening the vaginal entrance both experience extra stimulation.

BELOW RIGHT
Another Kama classic, the 'position of Indrani', allows the man very deep penetration but restricts his pace, so ensuring slower lovemaking.

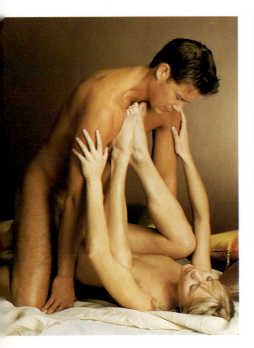

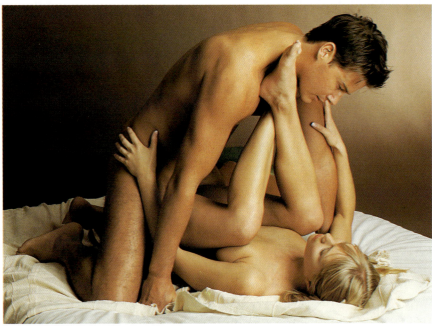

MAN-ON-TOP VARIATIONS   81

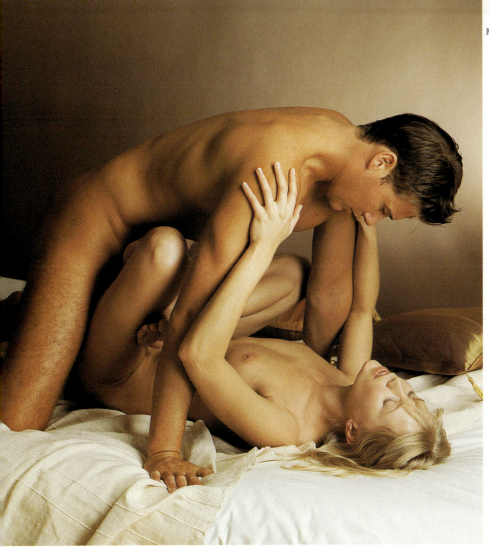

LEFT
In this Kama Sutra variation, his partner's legs are crossed in the lotus position and pressed back against her. It allows a change of penetration angle and a novel stimulus for both of them.

With flowers in her hair hanging loose, and her smiles broken by hard breathing, she should press upon her lover's bosom with her own breasts, and ... should say, 'I was laid down by you, and fatigued with hard congress, I should now therefore lay you down in return'.

describes this as the 'pressed position'. In this pose, the vaginal entrance is tighter, which increases the friction and, hence, the stimulation. The man can move only slowly in this position, so extending lovemaking. In the 'half-pressed position', one leg is compressed with the foot against the man's chest and the other leg is held out straight. The 'position of Indrani' (wife of the god Indra) is similar to the 'pressed position', but requires more flexibility on the part of the woman. As before, her feet are together and pressed against the man's chest but her knees are apart and her thighs are pressed back on either side of her body. This puts the man in total control, and so is best for loving, trusting and committed relationships only.

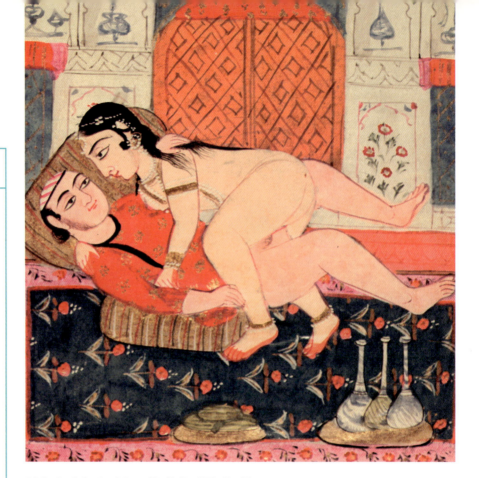

ASSERT YOURSELF

The days are long gone when females need be bashful about taking the lead. That said, not all women feel they can assert themselves during sex and direct the action. The 'woman-on-top position' offers the ideal opportunity to do just that. Here, the roles of control are reversed, and it is the man who must surrender to you. You decide how to proceed, while your partner lies supine beneath you. And you don't need to tell him in advance: let it be a great surprise or wrestle him for the privilege of being on top (but make sure you win!). Any reluctance on his part will fade once he discovers the new sensations he can experience now that you are the boss and dictating the moves.

WOMAN ON TOP

Vatsyayana didn't believe a man should be in total control during sex, or do all the work. He heartily recommends a woman climbing atop her lover, at the beginning or mid-way through lovemaking, to *'satisfy the curiosity of her lover, or her own desire of novelty'*. He also suggests the woman-on-top position when her lover is *'fatigued by constant congress'*. It is a simple matter for a woman to straddle her partner and then lower herself, slowly guiding his penis into her as she does so. The feeling of being in charge during intercourse is a major turn-on for a woman. She controls the pace and depth of penetration, and directs his penis to where she wants it. For extra stimulation, she can reach down to rub her clitoris and labia (or let her partner do it), while he fondles her breasts or strokes her buttocks and thighs. They can maintain eye contact throughout and continue to kiss and caress.

WOMAN-ON-TOP VARIATIONS

The easiest position to adopt is with the man lying on his back, legs straight, while his partner sits astride him with her knees on either side. By leaning forward to support herself on her hands, the woman can raise and lower herself on her partner's penis, taking as long as she likes to become fully aroused (he's not going anywhere) and then increasing the pace, if she chooses, as she approaches orgasm. By stretching out on top of him she can enhance the skin-to-skin contact, or move sinuously from side to side to increase the range of sensations. Alternatively, she can lean right back, again supporting herself on her hands, and place her feet on her lover's shoulders, rocking backwards and forwards to stimulate the G-spot on the front wall of her vagina. In this way she is using her partner as a sex toy – but he is not likely to mind that.

She can also turn the tables on the man by trying the 'pressed position' in reverse. This time the man keeps his knees and legs together and places his feet against her chest. With her knees either side of his waist, penning him in, and his knees pressed back into his chest, the woman has almost complete control. By combining this with bondage fantasy play (see pages 102–3), the man becomes her (willing!) sex slave.

Different kinds of congress, performed according to the usage of each country, and the liking of each individual, generate love, friendship and respect in the hearts of women.

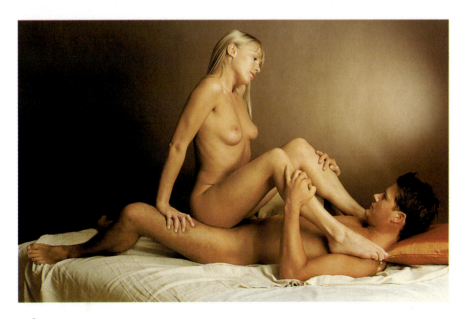

LEFT

In the on-top position, a woman is in total control. With her feet on her man's shoulders she can rock gently for slow, sensual G-spot stimulation.

SIDE BY SIDE

This is the most relaxed, affectionate and, perhaps, emotionally satisfying position for sex, when a couple have all the time in the world to show their feelings for one another. It is difficult to beat unhurried side-by-side lovemaking, alternating thrusting movements with spells of kissing and caressing. In this position it is easy to entwine arms and legs, stroke your partner's back, thighs and buttocks, gaze into each other's eyes and utter tender words, thereby enhancing the feeling of being loved, wanted and secure in your partner's embrace.

The pace and intensity of intercourse is shared, so neither lover is solely in control. Although there is less manoeuverability in this position than in most, that can be an advantage as it helps a man to control his arousal and delay climax. From lying side by side, it's simple to roll into the man- or woman-on-top positions to increase the pace.

SIDE-BY-SIDE VARIATIONS

Couples often move into the side-by-side position at the start of lovemaking, after an extended spell of petting and foreplay, or towards the end, to extend intercourse or when fatigue is starting to take hold. As the couple lie facing, the woman simply lifts her upper leg and places it over her partner's waist. If the man lies a little lower than his partner, he can easily push upwards to enter her. She can then keep her lower leg straight or slide her leg under his waist. Alternatively, she can place her lower leg between his legs so that they lay

An ingenious person should multiply the kinds of congress after the fashion of the different kinds of beasts and birds.

> **STAY IN TOUCH**
>
> **When making love it is important to continue to caress each other. This adds to the stimulation and hence the pleasure, and strengthens a couple's feelings for one another. Some positions, such as side by side and rear entry, enable men and women to caress parts of the body that are less accessible in other poses. The spine, in particular, is very sensitive, and lovers should take time to find the most erogenous areas. For men, the base of the spine is particularly arousing, whereas for women, it may be the neck, between the shoulder blades or the lower back. When lying side by side, couples can caress the buttocks, gliding a loving hand around and between the cheeks to stroke and squeeze or running a fingertip lightly around the anus, a bonus for men and woman.**

SIDE-BY-SIDE VARIATIONS 85

entwined. In this position, her legs are not open very wide, so the vagina remains quite tight, increasing the stimulation. By leaning away from each other they can alter the angle of penetration. If she chooses, the woman can wrap her legs around her partner's chest, or lift them up even further to encircle his neck. Or they could reverse roles, and the man can place his legs around those of his partner.

BELOW

Side-by-side positions offer opportunity for slow, languid, sensual sex. By altering her leg position, she can vary sensations.

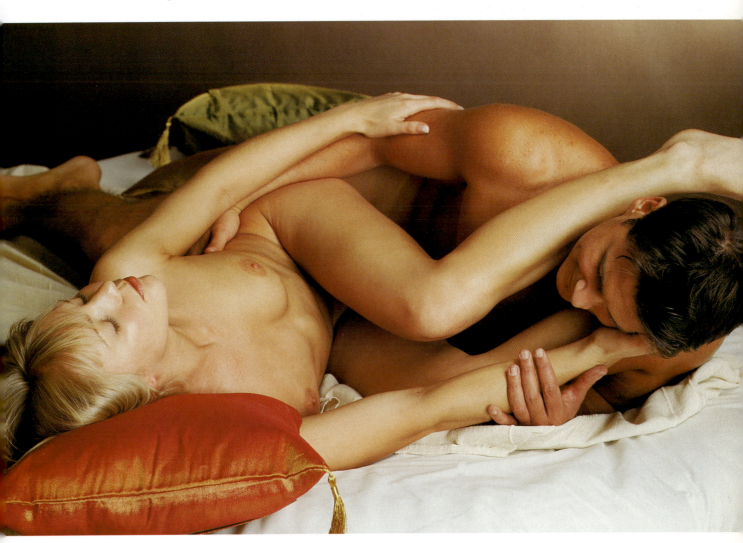

REAR-ENTRY SEX

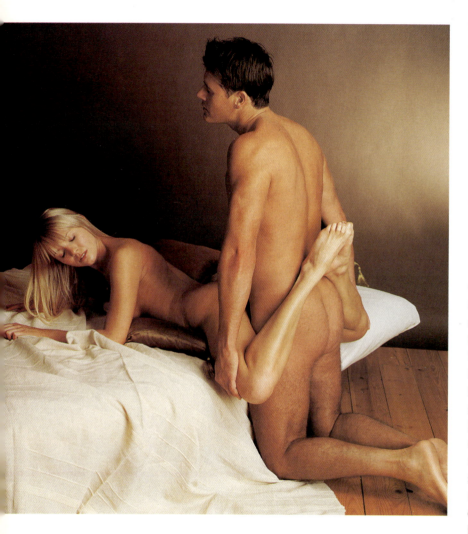

ABOVE
This rear-entry allows the woman to hook her feet around her partner for a close hold while he enters.

When a man penetrates his partner while he is behind her it is called rear-entry sex, or sometimes 'doggy style'. The Kama Sutra has many names for this position, including *'congress of a cat, cow, deer, dog or goat', 'forcible mounting of an ass', 'jumping of a tiger', 'pressing of an elephant', 'rubbing of a boar',* or *'mounting of a horse',* depending on the animal being emulated. *'In all these cases the characteristics of these different animals should be manifested by acting like them,'* Vatsyayana says.

Rear-entry sex can be performed when a couple are standing, kneeling, lying down, side by side or with a woman sitting astride her partner – but facing towards his feet. Indeed, if a woman turns round while her partner's penis is inside her, she can switch from face-to-face to rear-entry sex. Rear-entry offers a whole new range of sensations for both partners. For the man, it offers deeper penetration and a sense of novelty. Also, he is in a good position to stroke his partner's breasts, pubic mound, labia and clitoris to give her extra stimulation. For the woman, the benefits are that his penis is rubbing against a different area of her vagina and her sensitive buttocks are more directly in contact with his thrusts. She, too, can easily reach her pubic mound, labia and clitoris in this position. Although rear-entry is a fairly passive position for a woman, compared with woman-on-top and side-by-side, she can raise her buttocks and push back to synchronize with her partner's actions.

REAR-ENTRY VARIATIONS

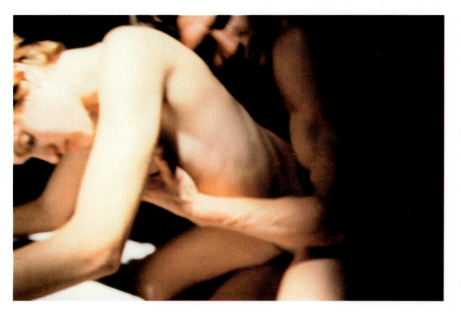

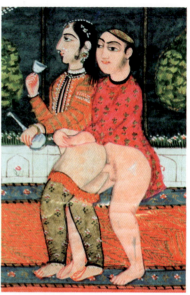

The man should gather from the action of the woman what things would be pleasing to her during congress.

Depending on the mood, rear-entry sex can be adventurous or relaxed. For example, the woman can remain standing and simply bend over and grip her ankles for support or hold on to a chair. Alternatively, she can support herself on hands and knees and her partner can kneel behind her. A more comfortable position for a woman is to lie on her front on the bed with her feet on the floor. Her partner then stands between her parted thighs and in this position can lift her legs slightly to change the angle of entry. For a more relaxed pose, rear-entry sex can be combined with side-by-side. This position is called 'spoons' because the bodies fit together so snugly. With the man's arms enfolding his partner in a loving embrace, this pose allows for relaxed and emotionally satisfying sex. The man can nuzzle his lover's neck and stroke her breasts and abdomen. After they have climaxed, the two lovers can drift off to sleep in a state of postcoital bliss.

ABOVE LEFT

From behind, a man is well placed to reach around to squeeze and fondle his lover's breasts, and to stroke her inner thighs and vulva to help her climax.

SEATED SEX

Seated sex can take many forms, such as sitting facing each other on the bed, with legs and arms entwined. Perhaps wrapped in your lover's lap while ensconced in an armchair in front of an open fire, maybe perched on the back seat of a car or parked in a secluded spot. Seated sex offers lots of scope for the imagination. While seated, a couple can gaze lovingly into each other's eyes, or kiss tenderly or passionately, or just take it easy, resting their heads together, making their lovemaking last as long as possible. Also, the hands are left free to explore each other's body.

The seated position is ideal for spontaneous sex, too. After a lengthy session of heavy petting on the sofa, once a woman is feeling really aroused she can take the initiative by climbing onto her partner's lap and wrapping her legs around him. They don't even need to strip off. The man simply unzips his flies, while his partner raises her skirt and slips her underwear down her thighs. For a woman, seated sex offers many advantages. The man's freedom of movements are limited, so he must keep his actions slow and steady, making it easier to extend lovemaking. Meanwhile, she can rock back and forth, controlling the pace and depth of penetration. She can change the angle of entry by wrapping her arms around his neck and pulling herself towards him, or leaning back to support herself with her hands, resting them on the floor or gripping his ankles.

FAR RIGHT

Seated sex is great for close, intimate touches and gentle caresses – combined with passionate kisses, to strengthen the emotional bond.

BELOW RIGHT

With their limbs entwined and bodies pressed close together, the seated position allows couples to begin their lovemaking slowly, tenderly ...

BELOW LEFT

... and steadily build to wild, energetic, abandoned sex, staying seated or rolling into one of the other positions to finish in a passion-fuelled frenzy.

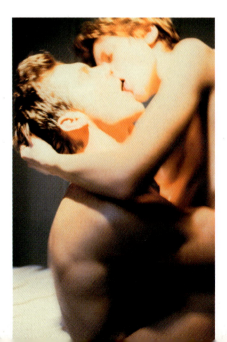
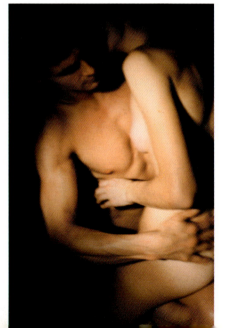

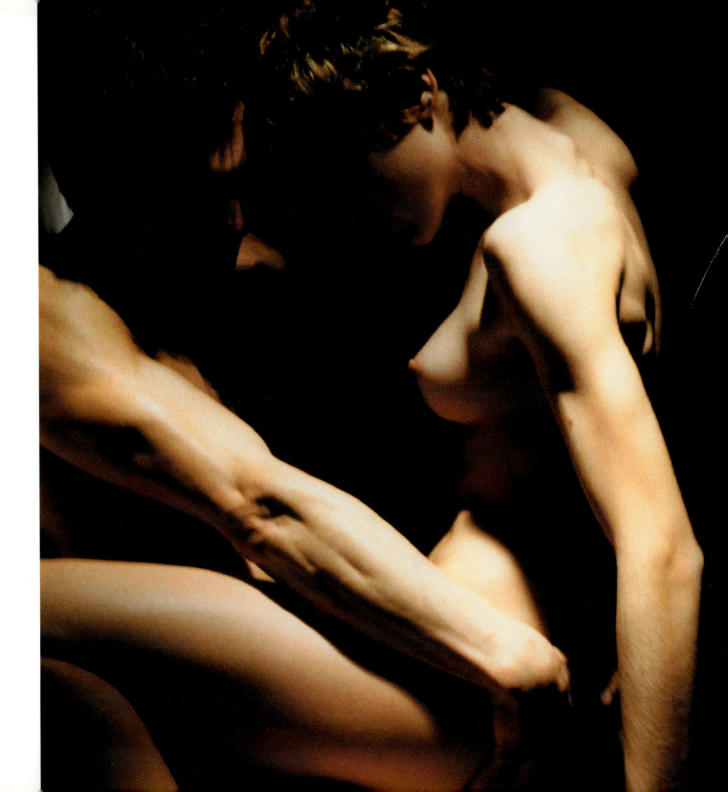

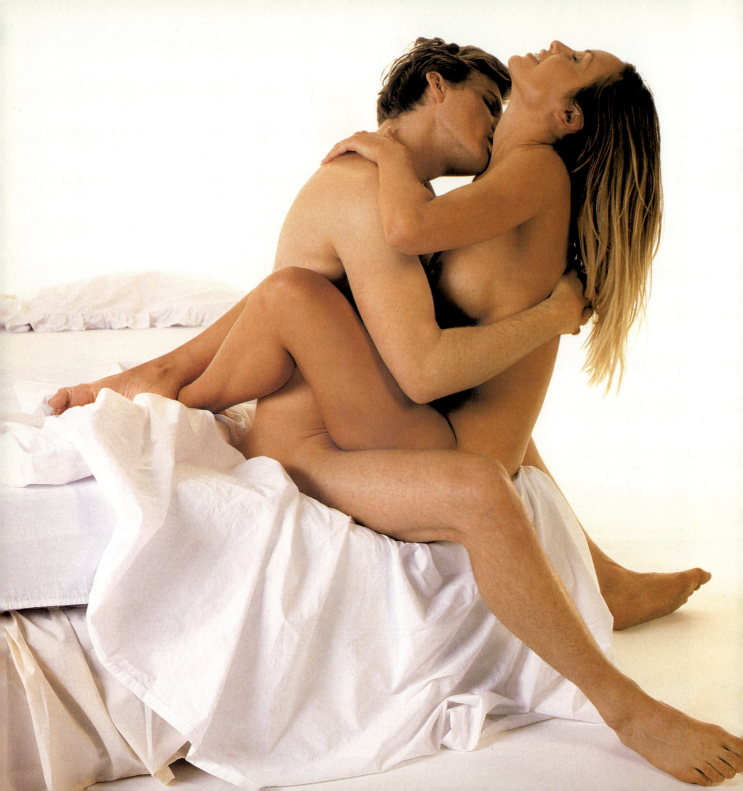

SEATED-SEX VARIATIONS

Sitting upright on the bed, a couple can entwine their legs for slow, sensual, loving sex. This pose is often adopted in Tantric sex (see pages 111–3). From this position, they can place their hands behind them on the bed and lean back as far as they like – even lying flat, if they choose. In an armchair, the man can sit back while his partner climbs aboard, placing her knees on either side of his upper body. This is like the woman-on-top position, so she is in control and the man has little to do other than use his mouth to good effect on his partner's neck, chest, breasts and nipples. A couple can combine their seated position with rear-entry sex, too. Here, the woman sits back onto the man's lap while he is sitting in the chair. She lowers herself onto him and either keeps her feet on the floor or places them on her partner's feet or legs.

STANDING SEX

This is a position for spontaneous moments of overwhelming passion when a couple simply cannot wait but must make love where they stand, her underwear discarded and skirt raised, his trousers at 'half-mast'. Their arms are wrapped around each other in a powerful embrace, covering each other's faces in hungry kisses. It is pure animal passion, and if both are extremely sexually aroused, an exciting and liberating experience. But standing sex is not for the weak, the easily fatigued, the faint-hearted or those with a bad back. In fact, in all its many forms, standing sex may be the most physically demanding of all the sex positions.

FAR LEFT
The Kama Sutra describes this intimate pose as the 'milk and water' embrace, as the two bodies melt into each other as if mingling to become a single substance.

When a man and woman enter into each other's bodies while the woman is sitting on the lap of the man, or on a bed, it is an embrace like the mixture of milk and water.

STANDING-SEX VARIATIONS

The Kama Sutra calls standing sex 'supported congress' and describes one form in which the man supports himself against a wall. *'The woman, sitting on his hands joined together and held underneath her, throws her arms around his neck, and putting her thighs alongside his waist, moves herself by her feet, which are touching the wall against which the man is leaning.'*

If the man has to support his partner's full weight, it may well help if he supports himself against *'a wall, or pillar'*. But this is not the only method. The woman can simply lift one leg, which her partner grips with one hand, while placing his other hand firmly behind her back to hold her steady. She can hold him firmly with one arm around his neck and the other about his waist. This position is easiest if the woman has long legs, relative to her partner. Otherwise he has to bend his knees to enter her, a difficult pose to maintain unless he is very fit. As Vatsyayana describes, the man can also link his hands to form a seat for his partner. The woman can then raise her other leg to grip her lover around his waist. Alternatively, he can support her legs under the thighs. In this pose, she can raise and lower her body in time with his pelvic thrusts. If she is flexible, she can lean back and support her weight by placing her hands on the floor.

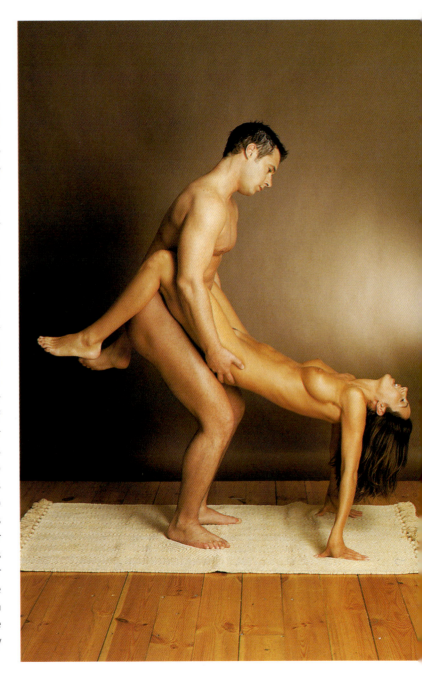

ADVENTUROUS SEX

You might think standing sex was adventurous enough, but the Kama Sutra has more suggestions to spice up your sex life. These positions involve an element of risk, unless both partners are fit, flexible – and careful. Before you experiment, it is wise to scatter pillows and cushions liberally on the floor around the bed, in case you fall off. If you do decide to try adventurous sexual positions, take it slowly, or you increase the risk of injury. Much of the fun comes from the time it takes to adopt the pose, with the book spread out before you, trying to work out how the couple in the picture managed to link up like that. If the only result is that you and your partner end up in a heap, giggling like schoolchildren, that's good too. Laughter is often a prelude to the best sex of all.

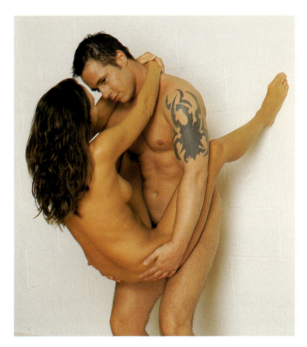

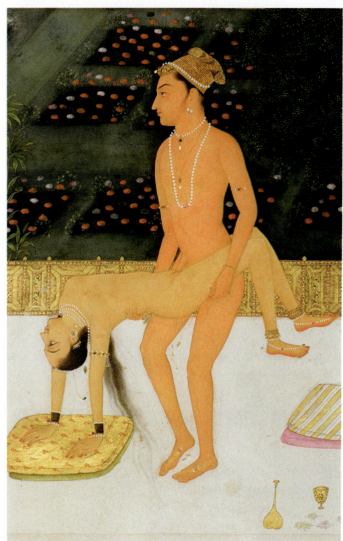

FAR LEFT
In this advanced standing pose, the woman leans back to support herself on the floor with her hands.

LEFT
'Supported congress' allows a woman to use the wall to raise her legs, while the man forms a seat with his hands.

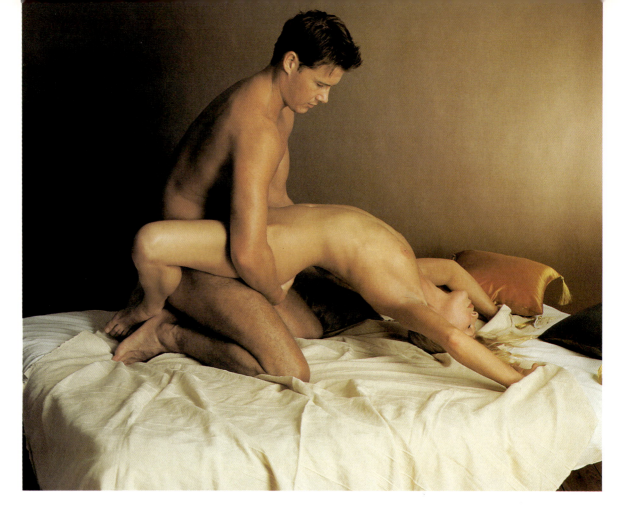

ADVENTUROUS SEX VARIATIONS

ABOVE
In the 'widely opened position', the woman arches her back into the shape of a bow, while he rocks back and forth.

FAR RIGHT
This combines standing and rear-entry sex. The woman grips her partner with her legs for support.

The possibilities for adventurous sex are limited only by your imagination – and the flexibility of your spine. As a test of both, the Kama Sutra suggests the 'widely opened position', also known as 'the bow', because of the shape the woman's body adopts. The man squats on the bed (or floor) and his partner lowers herself onto his penis, with her weight on her feet. She then leans right back until her head is touching the bed and begins to rock backwards and forwards, supporting herself on feet, hands and head (for a woman, the sensation is enhanced by a rush of blood to the head). A variation of this is 'inverted sex' in which the woman lies over the edge of the bed with her head

ADVENTUROUS SEX VARIATIONS

touching the floor. Her partner remains on the bed, positioned between her parted thighs and supporting her firmly around the waist, taking care that she doesn't slide on to the floor.

New and powerful sensations can be generated if the position – and direction – are changed while keeping the penis inside the vagina (see 'Warning' below before you try this). Vatsyayana describes two such poses in the Kama Sutra, the 'turning position' and the 'spinning top'. In the first of these, the woman lies flat on her back and the man enters her, and then manoeuvres himself round until he is facing the opposite way, with his thighs either side of his partner's waist. The woman can raise her legs and grip his waist with her thighs, while placing her feet on his shoulder blades. At the same time, the man can thrust back into her, while she can press down on his back with her heels. The 'spinning top' is a variant of this. Here, the man lies on his back while his partner straddles him, taking his penis into her. The woman then spins round slowly, through 180 degrees, until facing the opposite way. She is well placed to move up and down or rock backwards and forwards, controlling the angle and pace of stimulation. From his vantage point, the man can enjoy a different view of his partner and can stroke her back and buttocks. Or he can sit up and reach round to squeeze her breasts, or stroke her pubic mound, labia and clitoris.

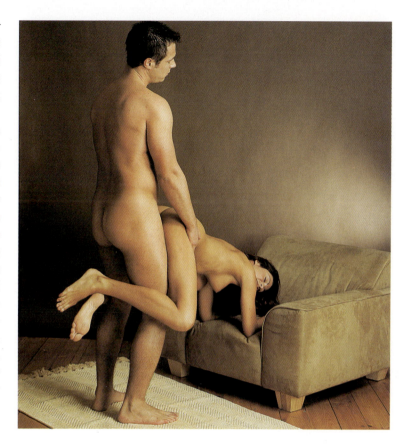

WARNING

Although the erect penis seems amazingly sturdy, it can be damaged. The erection is brought about by changes in blood flow: blood is pumped into the penis faster than it can be pumped away, causing the organ to swell. The penile blood vessels are under huge hydraulic pressure at this time, and may break if the organ is bent at too sharp an angle. Therefore, any twisting and turning movements by either partner while the penis is inside the vagina, should be carried out slowly and carefully. You must stop at once if there is pain or discomfort.

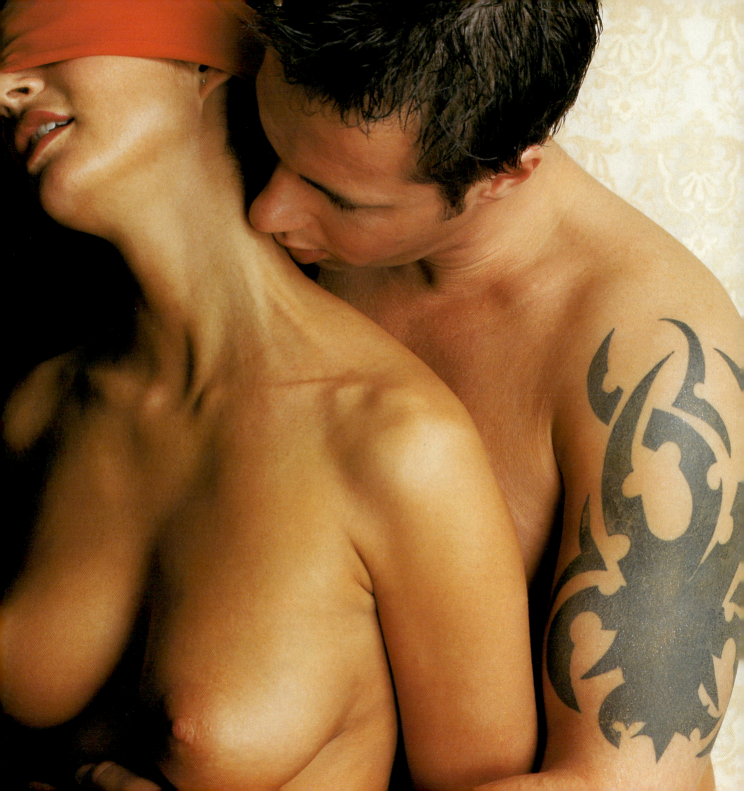

SEXUAL MAGIC

Such passionate actions and amorous movements, which arise on the spur of the moment and during sexual intercourse, cannot be defined and are as irregular as dreams.

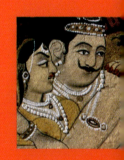

Once the heat of early romance dies down to the warm glow of long-term relationship, passion may cool a little. Even the most intensely loving partnership can lose its spark and may benefit from a liberal sprinkling of sexual magic to re-ignite the flames. Sex games put the fun back into foreplay, enliven lovemaking and revive the vibrancy of early courtship. Vatsyayana understood this well and stocked the Kama Sutra with lovers' games to spice up sex play.

A simple approach is to change location – having sex on the kitchen table or in the bath. If risk-taking is your thing, consider *al fresco* fun – making love on a moonlit lawn, or curled up on the back seat of a car parked in a secluded lovers' lane (but keep your doors locked, and bear in mind that it could be against the law, depending on where you live). Another way to enhance the erotic mood is through fantasy. Here, couples adopt sexy roles or act out arousing scenarios. Possibilities are limited only by your imagination. The ideas given here are meant to whet your appetite for experiment and encourage inventiveness.

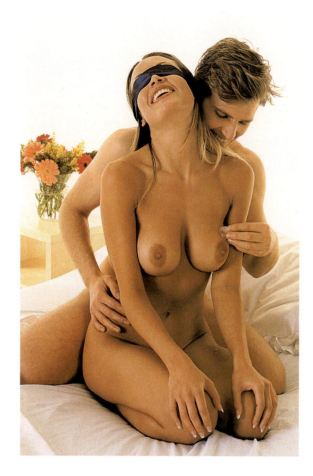

Congress having once commenced, passion alone gives birth to all the acts of the parties.

The Kama Sutra explores the link between pain and pleasure in mild sado-masochistic practices such as biting, scratching and smacking. But you may like to extend play to bondage or discover the delights of sex toys and props. Before we go any further, a warning. There's an element of risk in any sex game, and this is what makes it exciting. But this is fun – nothing more. You are playing in an erotic wonderland. It is not a test of your partner's courage or pain threshold, or an opportunity to settle old scores. Also, it's a natural female tendency to want to please her man, but women shouldn't feel obliged to do things they don't want to. You can get carried away, and may harm your health – and relationship. So, set strict ground rules in advance (see below).

SAFETY DOS AND DON'TS

Before contemplating any risky sex act, bear in mind the following:

- **Do** ensure that fastenings used in bondage can be loosened quickly and easily at any time by either partner.
- **Do** insist that smacking, scratching, biting and so on cause little more than mild pain.
- **Don't** attempt a physically demanding position or activity unless you know that you and your partner are fit enough, strong enough and flexible enough to cope.
- **Don't** undertake any sexual activity under the influence of drink or drugs.
- **Don't** agree to (or coerce a partner into) anything that risks severe pain or damage.
- **Don't** consider any activity involving pain or physical constraint unless you are in a relationship with someone you know well, love unconditionally and trust absolutely.

FANTASYLAND

Fantasy role play with a partner adds a new dimension to sex. By harnessing the power of the mind you become more easily aroused and maintain this heightened state throughout lovemaking. Studies show women enjoy sex more if they fantasize about it beforehand. Fantasy lets couples talk over and act out their innermost sexual desires. You might imagine making love on an ornate four-poster bed, or in a sun-kissed wooded glade, on a golden sandy beach, or in a luxury swimming pool. The options are endless. The Kama Sutra is packed with erotic imagery: ecstatic sex in an exotic palace garden, the scent of orange blossom wafting on the breeze, orgasmic cries mingling with the call of peacocks. In Vatsyayana's day, this was not fantasy, but how the nobility lived! Don't forget the concubines, highly trained in all the arts of sexual pleasure-giving. Wealthy women, too, had their sex slaves; men whose only role in life was to keep their mistresses satisfied. Keeping that thought in mind may energize your sexual imagination.

Clothes add an extra dimension to sexual fantasies. Their power lies not just in the touch and feel of certain fabrics and materials, although that is important. Clothes are powerfully evocative, reminding lovers of past moments of passion, or of screen and music idols that first aroused their sexual longings. Some clothes, such as lacy underwear, see-through shirts and blouses, tight trousers, boxer shorts or miniskirts, can be kept for intimate moments. Store in a dressing-up chest with items such as a military uniform, nurse's outfit and fireman's helmet, and don them to make your next fantasy more realistic.

Have a sexy cinema evening, and take the place of your screen idols in an erotic movie scene: Liza Minnelli sizzling in fishnet stockings and suspenders in *Cabaret*, Demi Moore and Patrick Swayze getting down and dirty as they shape pots in *Ghost*, Jessica Lange and Jack Nicholson battering the bakeware in *The Postman Always Rings Twice*. Immerse yourself in the role, really let go, and give an Oscar-winning performance. Staying with the film theme, in *Nine ½ Weeks*, Kim Basinger and Mickey Rourke famously frolicked with food – and you can do the same. Take turns to be blindfolded while your partner teases you with tasty morsels – never knowing what you'll get next. Experiment with different temperatures (warm chocolate, say, and ice cream), or tastes, (syrup followed by lemon). Pour honey or anything gooey on your partner's back, breasts/chest or thighs and lick it off, ever so slowly. Or take a mouthful of ice cream and a mouthful of your lover and see the electric effect this can have.

FAR LEFT

With eyes blindfolded, you can focus all your senses on your partner's touch – as he finds imaginative ways to arouse you.

BELOW

Sex in the open air is exciting – and very risky! Try it if you dare, or simply share an al fresco fantasy.

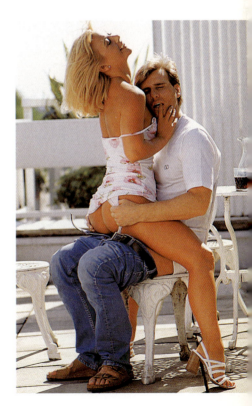

WATER WARNING

Because condoms may be ineffective in water, avoid making love in water if you are practising safer sex or if condoms are your only means of contraception. Water can be a dangerous medium to use in sex play so always use common sense.

- **Never submerge your lover's head, or place him or her in a position where this might happen by accident. (It is possible to drown in just a few inches of water.)**
- **Never direct a strong jet of water into any bodily orifice, such as mouth, ears, vulva or anus, as this can have potentially fatal consequences.**
- **Never use any electrical equipment near water or with wet hands.**

SEX GAMES

Erotic games are a great way to take the performance pressure out of lovemaking and make sex more fun. Find ideas that offer opportunities for undressing, touching, fondling and groping. Sex shops sell games for this very purpose, or contact games such as 'Twister' give couples lots of chances to get intimate. Strip poker is the best-known sexy card game, in which you bet items of clothing instead of money, but you can adapt any card game, with the loser paying a forfeit. You might have to remove a clothing item, or lie perfectly still while an intimate part of your body is stroked, squeezed or sucked. Or the punishment for a run of bad luck might be to masturbate your partner, or give or receive oral sex – unlucky in cards really does mean lucky in love[making].

WATER PLAY

Water is a versatile medium that can enrich your love life. In the bath or shower, cover your lover's skin with rich, soapy lather and gently stroke and massage the flesh. Soap lubricates the skin, allowing your hands to glide over its surface. Or rub a loofah or flannel briskly over the skin to make the nerve endings tingle. Rinse off by pouring water over your lover's body in cascading rivulets. Or use a hand-held shower attachment to direct a light jet of water onto different areas of the body – over breasts, nipples and genitals for powerfully arousing sensations. The warm, soothing water is not just removing soap but also washing away cares and tensions. If your passion surfaces in the bath, don't spoil the moment by getting out to dry off – just straddle your partner and make love there. The friction of wet clinging skin between your writhing bodies enhances the erotic enjoyment.

BAWDY GAMES **Board games can become bawdy games simply by changing the penalties. In Monopoly, for example, instead of paying rent when you land on an occupied square, remove – or wear – an item of clothing of your partner's choice. Create your own 'community chest' cards, each one featuring a different sex-related activity, to be carried out whenever it turns up. The suspense element adds to the enjoyment – as you wait for the roll of the dice to reveal who'll do what, to whom – and when.**

WATER PLAY

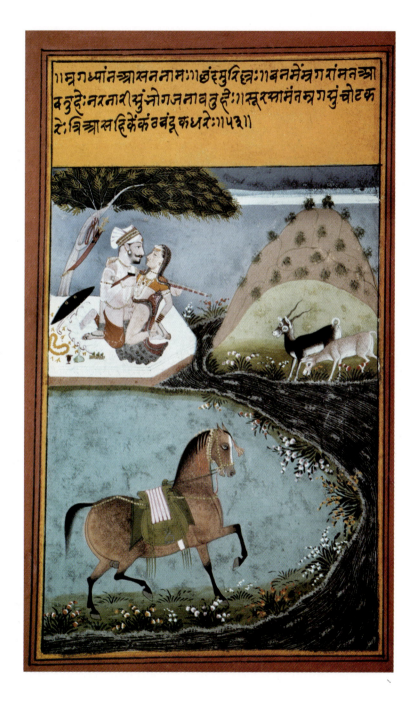

A horse, having once attained the fifth degree of motion, goes on with blind speed, regardless of pits, ditches and posts in the way. In the same manner, a loving pair become blind with passion in the heat of congress, and go on with great impetuosity, paying not the least regard to excess.

DOMINATION AND BONDAGE

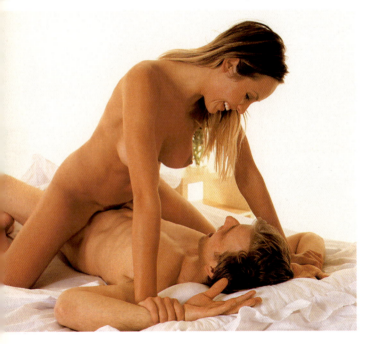

FAR RIGHT
Power games allow you to express a hidden side of your nature.

BELOW
Taking a dominant role can be a turn-on for a woman, as she forces her helpless partner to submit to her carnal desires.

Fantasy games of domination and bondage are always popular, and it's easy to see why. They allow couples to adopt new bedroom personae, far removed from their day-to-day character. Shy, retiring types can take command and reveal their more dominant side. Those who make decisions all day long can relinquish responsibility and give in to a lover's whims and fancies. If you are in charge, the sense of sexual power you feel can electrify your lovemaking. And if you are the submissive one, being enslaved by a lust-crazed lover releases you from all responsibility – and guilt – and allows your innermost sexual desires to bubble to the surface.

Domination involves total control over your lover, forcing him or her to submit to your will. In a typical dominatrix session, a woman, for example, will dress in knee- or thigh-length leather boots, with extra-high heels, and carry a whip or stick with which she imposes discipline. The slave is skimpily dressed, perhaps in a thong, or naked except for dog collar and/or manacles, to reinforce his servile role. The dominatrix orders him to carry out menial tasks that establish her authority and his lowly status, accompanied by demeaning phrases such as 'you are a miserable, feeble, pathetic worm who is not fit to lick my boots' (while ordering him to lick her boots). She threatens severe discipline unless the slave satisfies her every desire, and may administer the occasional slap or (gentle) flick of the whip. The dominant partner can be as insulting as he or she likes, just so long as the terms are non-specific. For example, it is fine to say your partner is 'as worthless as the dust beneath my feet', but resist the temptation to add 'and you're a rubbish driver, too', which might be taken personally.

Once you have established your dominant status, you can order your slave to perform – or submit to – a sex act of your choice. The theme can be adapted to a fantasy scenario, such as 'headmistress and naughty schoolboy', 'prisoner and warder', or 'lord of the manor and scullery maid'.

Bondage games are a type of domination. The mild form most commonly practised is called 'vanilla'. Typically, one person's wrists are tied behind their back or secured at the head of the bed while the other partner takes advantage of their lover's confined position to carry out a teasing form of sexual 'torture'. Anything that can be tied can be used to bind your lover, but ideally choose soft, non-chafing materials such as a silk scarf or ribbons, strips of velvet or brushed cotton. Sex shops stock specialist restraints such as soft bondage ropes, fur-lined handcuffs, tape with Velcro fastening, or leather manacles. As this is an extension of fantasy play, you don't need to fasten the bonds tightly, a simple loop will do. Or tie a bow rather than a knot. To add to the 'victim's' feeling of helplessness, and to give extra scope for teasing, the bound partner may be blindfolded. He or she can't see what you're doing, so the erotic suspense is more intense.

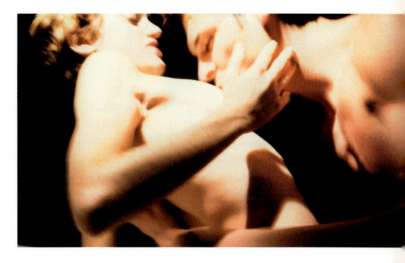

In surveys, lovemaking while a partner is tied is one of the most popular sexual fantasies revealed by men and women. The rules of the game depend on personal preference. Physical pain, unless it is mild, should be avoided. Otherwise, you are free to do whatever you please – and to take as long as you like doing it. For example, 'sensitize' your lover by running an ice cube over her breasts and abdomen, or stroke her thighs with a feather. Gently caress her body all over, running your hands over arms and shoulders, abdomen and legs, approaching breasts and vulva with agonizing slowness. Let her arousal build steadily, choosing the right moment to kiss and lick her body. If you are learning her responses, you'll know when to introduce teasing pauses, so that she begs you to keep going. A vibrator (see pages 109–10) applied to breasts and abdomen, along inner thigh and – especially – against her vulva, is exquisite torture in this position. Meanwhile, your partner can enter her own fantasy world (imagining you as an Oriental slave master, for example).

SEX GAME DOS AND DON'TS

Before taking part in sex games, set the rules in advance, and keep to them. For example:

- **Do agree on a code word or other signal that indicates your partner wants to stop (saying 'Please stop!' is no good if your partner thinks it's part of the game). Once the signal is given, stop immediately.**
- **Do decide whether pain is simulated or real. If the latter, agree the maximum level to be inflicted.**
- **Do ensure you can release yourself from ropes, chains, manacles and other restraints.**
- **Don't use force likely to inflict actual physical harm, such as bruising or cuts, or leave your partner in a situation where they may come to harm.**
- **Don't make personal remarks that might cause real offence or leave emotional scars.**
- **Don't play sex games following an argument or unresolved grievance against your partner.**

SMACKING, BITING AND SCRATCHING

WHIPPING UP FUN

For couples who wish to experiment with different forms of chastisement, there is a wide range of whips, flails, crops, paddles and lashings on offer. These inflict mild stinging rather than severe pain, spreading the sensation over a wider area. Start gently and gradually increase the strength until you find the level your partner 'likes' (or willingly tolerates). Alternate pain with tender touches. Contact should be made with broad or fleshy areas of the body only, nowhere near the face and eyes. As with spanking, props can be incorporated into fantasy and role-play.

Some people find that receiving and/or inflicting mild pain during sex greatly increases their pleasure. Others consider pain to be incompatible with lovemaking. The Kama Sutra caters for all tastes, so there are sections devoted to smacking, biting and scratching. However, Vatsyayana was opposed to any activity that may potentially cause severe pain, injury or scarring, calling such practices *'barbarous, and base, and quite unworthy of imitation'*. Pain sensitizes the nervous system, energizing nerve endings and the pathways that transmit sensory stimuli to the brain. The body then becomes more sensitive to erotic touch sensations. For best effect, follow each smack with caressing touches and kisses. To avoid injury, smacking should be applied only to fleshy areas of the body, principally thighs or buttocks, and administered with the flat of the fingers rather

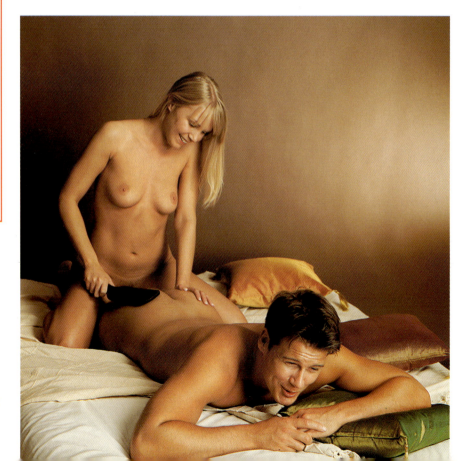

RIGHT
This is your chance to administer stern punishment for some offence, real or imagined – but remember, only in fun!

SMACKING, BITING AND SCRATCHING

than the palm of the hand. For men who relish being dominated (see above), a spanking given as punishment for a minor misdemeanor adds to the fantasy.

The Kama Sutra lists various forms of bite, distinguished mainly by the number of teeth used and the pattern they leave (see page 106). In Vatsyayana's day, a lover's bite mark was a sign of affection and regard – a trophy to be paraded publicly. Today, a love bite on an exposed area of skin causes more embarrassment than pride. Yet a little teeth-inflicted pain in a hidden, fleshy area of the body can be arousing. The sense of being secretly 'branded' by a lover and therefore his or her 'property' helps to strengthen emotional bonds. This issue is highly personal, so say from the outset if biting appeals or not. Take care not to bite your lover so hard their skin is broken. 'Safer sex' rules (see page 120) apply to biting and scratching just as much as any other sexual activity.

In Vatsyayana's day, scratching with the nails was an art form, with highly descriptive names given to marks etched out on the skin of a loved one. Simple

She should take hold of her lover's hair, and bend his head down, and kiss his lower lip, and then, being intoxicated with love, she should shut her eyes and bite him in various places.

LEFT
Mild pain during sex can heighten the skin's sensitivity and make the gentle caresses that follow even more arousing.

KAMA BITING

The following are some of the bites described in the Kama Sutra:

- *Hidden bite* This is shown only by the excessive redness of the skin.
- *Swollen bite* The skin is pressed down on both sides.
- *Point* A small portion of the skin is bitten with two teeth only.
- *Line of points* Small portions of the skin are bitten with all the teeth.
- *Coral and jewel* Teeth and lips are brought together (lips are the coral, teeth the jewel).
- *Line of jewels* Biting is performed with all the teeth.
- *Broken cloud* An impression is left from a circular bite, arising from the marks of the teeth and the spaces between.

marks were lines, circles and half moons. A small, curved line was called a *'tiger's claw'*, while a curved mark made with five nails was called *'a peacock's foot'* and, we are told, *'requires a great deal of skill to make properly'*. Five marks made close to one another are *'the jump of a hare'*. A similar but more elaborate design was the *'leaf of the blue locust'*. But there was no need to leave a mark for it was possible to *'press the chin, breasts, the lower lip, or jaghana (abdomen) of another so softly that no scratch or mark is left, but only the hair on the body becomes erect from the touch of the nails, and the nails themselves make a sound'*. According to Vatsyayana, *'pressing with the nails is not a usual thing except with those who are intensely passionate'*.

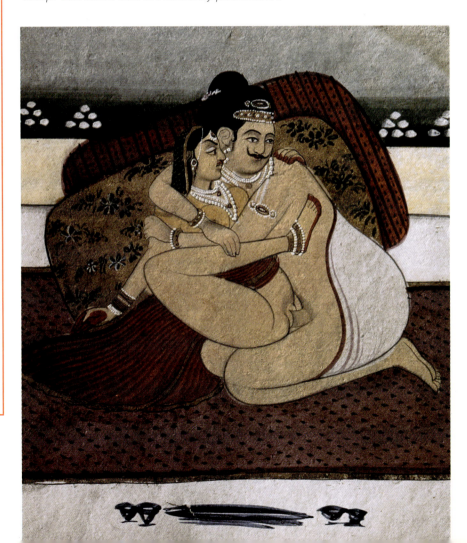

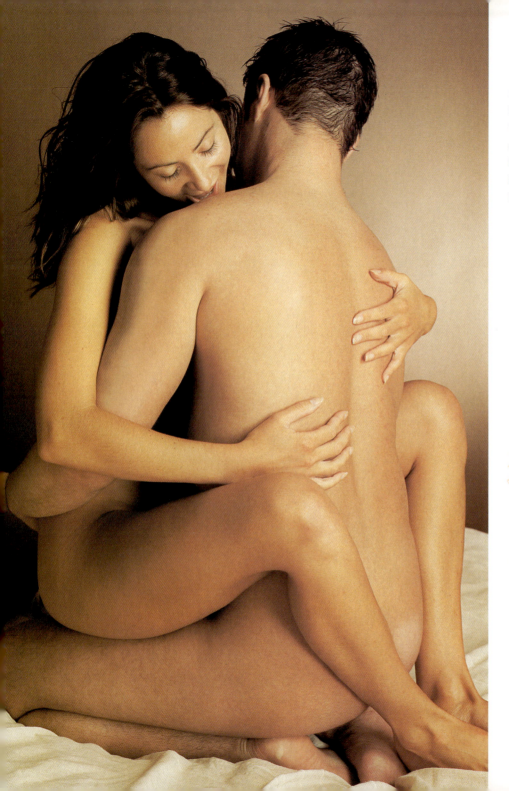

LEFT
In Vatsyayana's day, 'marking' your lover with a gentle bite mark at the height of passion was an intimate sign of the bond between you.

Even by day, and in a place of public resort, when her lover shows her any mark that she may have inflicted on his body, she should smile at the sight of it.

SEXUAL MAGIC

108

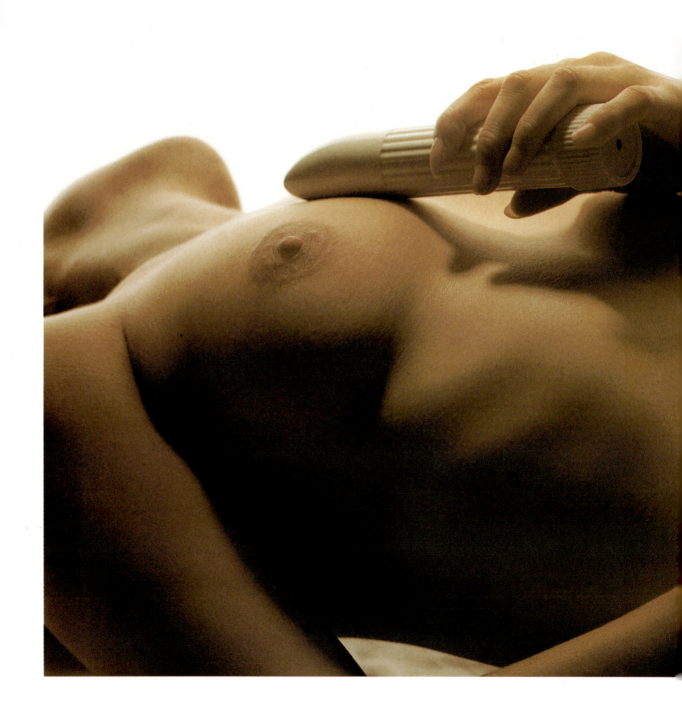

SEX TOYS

The best-known sex toy in Vatsyayana's day was the dildo, or artificial penis, crafted from polished ebony or ivory. This spiced up a couple's love life, or was employed by ladies of the harem on their days off. Dildos are still available as hand-held types or strap-ons to be worn around the waist but generally they have been superseded by the more popular, and versatile, vibrator. In effect a dildo with an electric motor whirring inside. The vibrations energize nerve endings not aroused by other forms of stimulation. The vibrator was originally marketed as a massage aid, for relaxation, and can be applied all over the body, especially on tense muscles and sensitive areas of skin – throat, breasts, abdomen and buttocks. Using a vibrator for the first time can be mind-blowing.

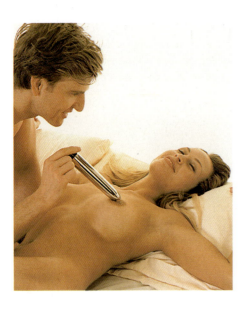

Many women get their most powerful orgasms by applying a vibrator to the vulva, perineum, clitoris or inside the vagina itself, especially to the G-spot. Men can enjoy arousing sensations created by a vibrator, not only when applied to the genitals but also when placed on the nipples, abdomen or perineum – indeed, everywhere!

There are many types (see right), some with sophisticated controls and variable settings. If using a vibrator for the first time, start on the lowest setting and slowly increase the speed until you find the sensation you prefer. Some small, oddly shaped devices do not look at all penile. These are designed to target specific parts of the body; some have a 'tongue action' to stimulate the clitoris, or a sharp bend to reach the G-spot. But they can often be used elsewhere on the body. Other devices, called 'love eggs', 'love balls' or 'magic bullets', are retained within the vagina. Made of smooth metal or spiny rubbery plastic, these include powered types, or solid ones designed to stimulate the vagina during rocking, or pelvic thrusting movements, with a partner or when 'flying solo'.

GOOD VIBRATIONS

If you haven't visited a sex shop recently you may be surprised at the range of vibrators on offer. The standard plain, white plastic type is still available – in various sizes. You can also buy vibrators that mimic a real penis – albeit, a generously proportioned one – even with lumps and veins. 'Fun' types are brightly coloured and made of soft, yielding, rubbery (and often flexible) plastic, with fins for extra stimulation. Waterproof types are for bath-time fun. Most vibrators have variable settings, and may rotate or move from side to side. Some, such as 'Jessica Rabbit', have attachments designed to stimulate the clitoris and/or anus at the same time.

LEFT
In the hands of a skilled lover, the vibrator can carry you to new heights – especially when applied to erogenous zones.

FAR LEFT
A vibrator can teach you about your body, and help you discover new areas of sensitivity for your partner to explore.

There are specialist devices for men, too, in the form of vibrating sleeves, into which the penis is inserted. 'Cock rings' and 'stud rings' fit around the erect penis, designed to hinder blood flow leaving the penis, so helping to maintain an erection. C-rings combine a cock-ring, to maintain his erection, and a vibrator, to stimulate her clitoris. Anal vibrators, as the name suggests, are inserted into the anus where – in men – they stimulate the prostate gland. This walnut-sized gland, which produces seminal fluid, lies next to the bladder and adjacent to the rectum. It has been called the 'male G-spot' as it produces powerful sexual feelings when stimulated, for example, during anal penetrative sex. The anus is not self-lubricating, unlike the vagina, and so anything inserted into it should be well lubricated with a suitable gel.

TOYS FOR BOYS – AND GIRLS

The following sex aids were developed for men, but women can have fun with them, too.

- *Nipple clamps* These cause mild pain to sensitize the nipples. Once the clamps are removed, the nipples are more responsive to pleasurable stimuli. As a woman's nipples are naturally highly sensitive, she may find the pain too intense to bear.
- *Butt plugs* Rubber or plastic plugs that are inserted into the anus. They can be left in place or moved around to increase the stimulus.
- *Pleasure beads* Strings of beads of tapering sizes that are inserted into the anus or vagina. They are then pulled out – slowly or quickly – during sex.

WARNING

Sex toys obtained from reputable suppliers are generally safe, but take precautions.

- Do wash sex toys after use, especially if used in or near the anus. Never insert any device into the vagina without first washing it.
- Do use lubricating gel with any device intended to be inserted into the anus.
- Don't use force to insert a device into any orifice.
- Don't share sex toys if your partner's sexual history is unknown. Alternatively, cover the toy with a condom, which you dispose of afterwards.
- Don't use any device designed to restrict blood flow from the penis without seeking your doctor's advice if you have an on-going medical condition, such as diabetes mellitus, heart or lung disease, high blood pressure or other circulatory problems.

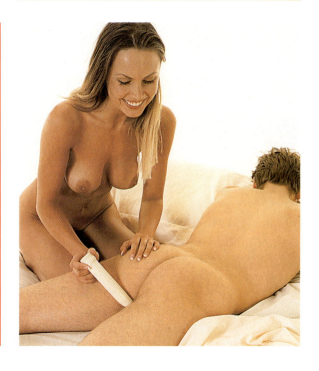

DIVINE SEX

To Westerners, there may seem no link between sex and religion. To ancient Indian cultures, however, the sex act was divine. The teachings of Vatsyayana and other scholars came to be incorporated into writings known as the Tantra. Tantrikas (followers of Tantra) sought to expand mental and spiritual consciousness through meditation, yoga, mantras and sex. Lovemaking is prolonged and orgasm delayed to harness sexual energy and use it to transport lovers to a higher plane of spirituality. Experienced couples can make love for hours. This is called 'riding the wave'.

Many people gain their first experience of Tantra through workshops where they receive instruction from an accredited teacher. But couples can experience the joys of Tantric sex by themselves. Even if you don't attain the dizzy heights achieved by Tantra devotees, you should still gain much from the experience, such as an enhanced relationship with a partner and better understanding of your lover's sexual needs. Choose a time when you can guarantee peace, quiet and freedom from interruptions. (Tell friends and relations you've gone away!) Create an Eastern mood with exotic aromas, beautiful ornaments and flowers. Place soft rugs, blankets and cushions on the floor. Feed each other exotic foods, ideally with aphrodisiac qualities (see page 37). Take turns to wash each other and then give each other a massage using scented oils (see pages 46–9) to create a relaxed, intimate mood. Let your hands explore all parts of your partner's body, finding new areas of sensitivity. By taking your time you can achieve a slow, sensual build-up.

You are now ready to begin. Sit facing each other as close as possible. Tantrikas adopt the cross-legged 'lotus' pose but it is more important to find one that is comfortable for you. Place your right palm over your partner's heart. He or she then places a hand over your heart. Breathe deeply into your abdomen, and gaze into your lover's eyes, focusing your thoughts exclusively on your partner. Concentrate on the rise and fall of your chest as you inhale and exhale, aiming to synchronize your breathing. Become aware of each other's heartbeat via your palms. As you relax, your heart rates will slow. Once you become emotionally more in tune, your heartbeat may match that of your partner.

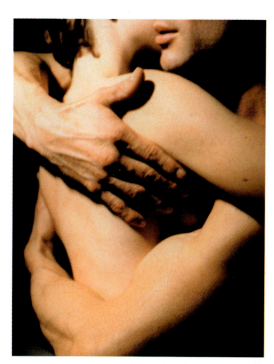

BELOW

'Divine' forms of sexual expression enable couples to attain a 'oneness' that can enhance all areas of their relationship.

FAR LEFT

In men, and women, the perineum – the area directly behind the genitals – is highly sensitive, especially when stimulated with a vibrator.

FAR RIGHT
Devotees of Tantric sex remain virtually still for long periods of time, using their 'fire (pelvic floor) muscles' to maintain a state of orgasmic bliss.

BELOW RIGHT
Any position that restricts the man's freedom of movement can be used to delay orgasm, and so allow couples time to seek a spiritual dimension to sex.

Now you are ready to make love. The aim of Tantric sex is to delay orgasm for as long as possible. This is easier for women, who generally take longer to climax. Therefore it is important to find a position that does not provide intense stimulation for the man. Seated positions (see pages 88–91) are ideal. The man sits cross-legged on the floor. His partner sits in his lap and entwines her legs around his waist. This position allows them to gaze into each other's eyes and focus their thoughts on each other. If the man becomes too aroused he should breathe more slowly and deeply to help delay his climax. The woman can contract her pelvic floor muscles around his penis (see page 24) to maintain his erection. Alternatively, he can lie on his back while his partner sits astride him (see pages 82–3), especially useful if he begins to tire. In this position, the woman can control the pace of lovemaking more easily.

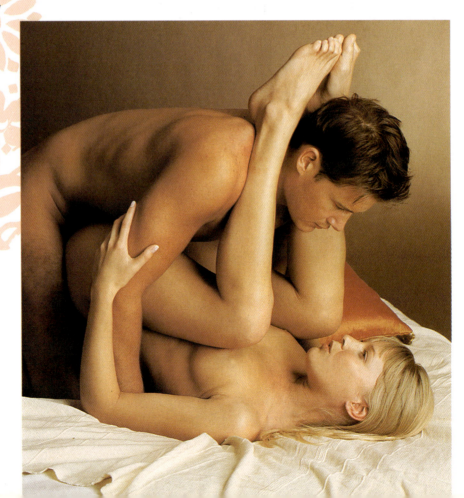

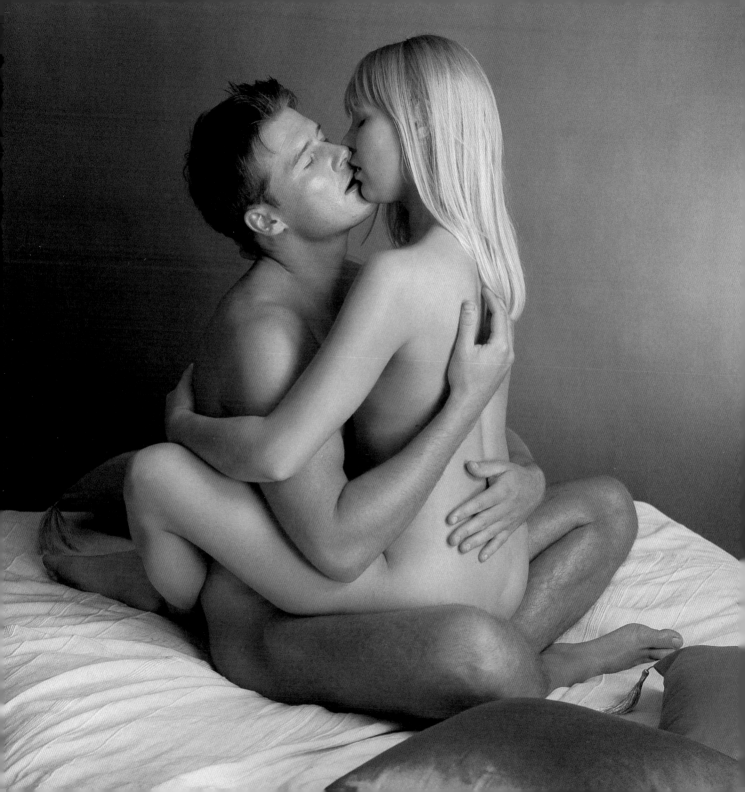

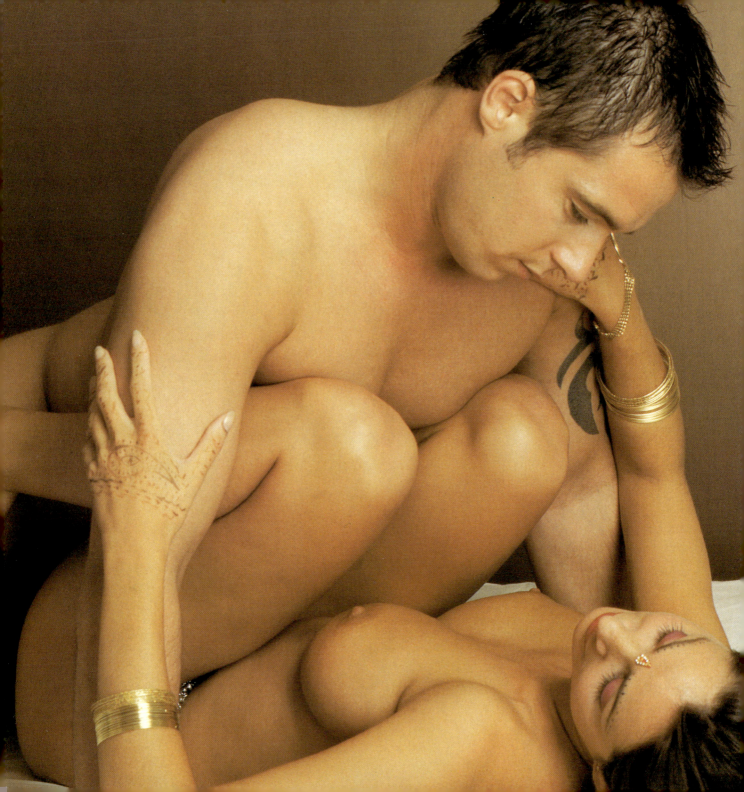

APPENDIX:
SAFETY ISSUES AND SEXUAL PROBLEMS

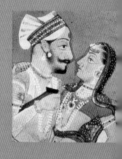

Sex is a fun game that adults play. But with the fun comes adult responsibilities, such as avoiding unplanned pregnancy, ensuring that you do not catch – or pass on – sexually transmitted infections (STIs), and staying out of danger. Be a 'good scout' and *be prepared:* hoping for the best but ready for the worst. If this seems alarmist, remember that most Western countries are seeing increases in unplanned pregnancies, STIs and sexual violence. Alcohol and drugs, taken voluntarily or without the person's knowledge, are often to blame. No one thinks it will happen to him or her, *until it does.* Yet this is not rocket science. There are basic steps everyone can take to stay safe.

At any time in a relationship sex problems can occur and should never be ignored. They may indicate an underlying physical disorder requiring treatment, or psychological or emotional factors that can put a relationship under strain. Most family doctors are trained to deal with sexual and relationship issues; specialists such as relationship counsellors and sex therapists can help too.

CONTRACEPTION

There is a wide range of methods available to prevent unplanned pregnancy; they fall into two main classes, barrier and hormonal. (The intra-uterine contraceptive device has elements of both and so is in a class of its own.) Barrier methods, such as male and female condoms, help protect against infection too. Your doctor can help you decide the best method for you, or talk to specialists at family planning/birth control clinics, who will have the latest information and can guarantee confidentiality. The reliability figures given below are based on the number of women out of 100 who might get pregnant if using a particular method for a year. As a guide, unprotected sex is only 20 per cent reliable; that is, 80 out of 100 women would become pregnant after a year of regular sex without contraception.

BARRIER METHODS

There are two main types of condom: one designed for men and one for women.

Male condom The only contraceptive now available for men (although birth control pills for males are being tested). It is a plastic (polyurethane) or rubber (latex) sheath that fits over the penis and prevents semen entering the vagina. The condom has a small bulb or teat at the tip that traps the semen. As soon as the man has ejaculated, he must withdraw his penis before he loses his erection, or the condom might slip off. He then disposes of the condom. Condoms are reliable (98–99 per cent), especially if combined with spermicide (but avoid those impregnated with nonoxynol-9, see Spermicide Safety, page 118). There is no stigma in a woman carrying condoms, so it makes sense for both men and women to keep condoms with them at all times, in a wallet or purse, if there is any chance of having sex, no matter how remote. Condoms can be tricky to use at first (see Fitting a Condom, opposite), so practise till perfect – before you need to fit one for real. While men can practise on themselves, women can use a banana or vibrator. By fitting a condom on her partner, a woman can make protection part of foreplay. He'll enjoy her touch and she can have fun teasing him.

Female condom Much larger than its male counterpart, the female condom is designed to line the vagina; a springy inner ring rests against the cervix (neck of the uterus) and an outer ring lies over the labia. Unlike the male condom, the female version can be left in place for a while after sex.

Diaphragm, cap and sponge These devices fit inside the vagina and prevent sperm from reaching an egg. They are used with a spermicide (see Spermicide Safety, page 118). A doctor or nurse, usually at a family planning/birth control clinic, is available to teach women how to fit them. The diaphragm covers the whole of the cervix while the cap just covers the cervical opening and is held there by suction. The sponge is liberally filled with spermicide and inserted into the vagina. The cap and diaphragm are reliable when used with spermicide (97–98 per cent) whereas the sponge is slightly less reliable (94–96 per cent).

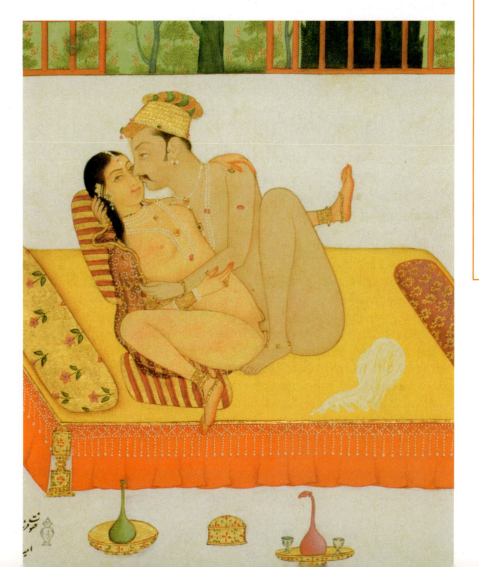

FITTING A MALE CONDOM

Avoid tearing a condom with nails or jewellery. If the condom gets damaged, throw it away and use another. To fit a condom:

1. Take the condom out of its package. Squeeze air out of the teat and place the condom on the tip of the erect penis.
2. Holding the teat, roll the condom down to the base of the penis, taking care not to stretch it too tightly.
3. After ejaculation, hold the base of the condom as the penis is withdrawn to prevent semen spilling out.
4. Peel off the condom, wipe the penis with a tissue and wrap the condom in the tissue before discarding it. Use a new condom for each act of intercourse.

RIGHT
For couples in monogamous relationships, hormonal methods of birth control are great for spontaneous – and worry-free – lovemaking.

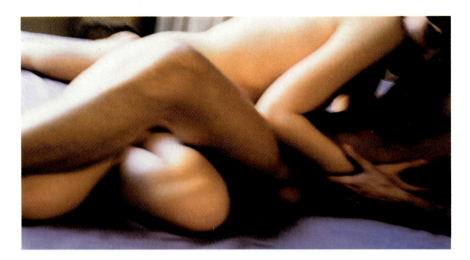

SPERMICIDE SAFETY

The use of a spermicide increases the efficacy of barrier methods. Ideally, spermicide is left in place for six hours after sex. The most widely used spermicide, nonoxynol-9, is best avoided in condoms and gels as it may increase the risk of contracting HIV. Its use in spermicidal creams and gels for caps, diaphragms and sponges is considered safe for women in monogamous relationships. It can cause skin irritation.

HORMONAL METHODS

Using oestrogen and/or progestogen, hormonal methods are designed to duplicate some of the physical changes that take place in a pregnant woman's body, which inhibit conception. Hormonal methods may not be suitable for older or overweight women, smokers or those with on-going medical conditions. Your doctor will advise. All hormonal methods are reliable (98–99 per cent for combined pill, injections and implants and 97–98 per cent for the mini-pill).

Combined pill and mini-pill These are the most widely used forms. The combined pill, containing oestrogen and progestogen, is usually taken for 21 days, followed by seven pill-free days or seven dummy pills. Other regimens also exist. The progestogen-only mini-pill (POP) must be taken every day within the same three-hour 'window' or protection may fail (see Pill Warnings, opposite).

Injectables and implants Long-term hormonal methods, injectables protect for two to three months. Implants are small capsules or rods inserted into the skin of the upper arm that protect for up to five years.

Morning-after pill Emergency contraception, used up to three days (ideally within 12 hours) of unprotected sex, or if a contraceptive method may have failed. Most family planning/birth control clinics recommend that women keep emergency contraception in hand as a back up. It should not be used as a regular form of contraception. Also, you should not put yourself at risk by having unprotected sex.

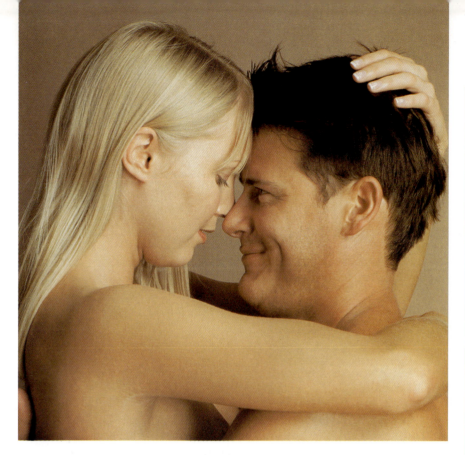

INTRA-UTERINE CONTRACEPTIVE DEVICE (IUCD)

This is a small T-shaped device that is inserted into the uterus and left in place for several years. It must be fitted and checked regularly by a doctor or other specialist. It is thought to work by making the uterus hostile to sperm, and by stopping a fertilized egg implanting in the wall of the uterus. Some types also release progestogen. The IUCD is reliable (97–98 per cent) but carries a slight risk of pelvic inflammatory disease (PID), infertility and ectopic pregnancy (where the foetus develops outside the uterus), and may not be suitable for all women. The risk is lower for women in monogamous relationships who have completed their families. Your doctor can advise. The IUCD is an effective means of emergency contraception, too, and can be fitted up to five days after unprotected sex (ideally, the sooner the better).

PILL WARNINGS

If you get into a routine of taking the pill at the same time each day, you're less likely to forget. This is essential with the progestogen-only mini-pill. If you do forget, take it as soon as you remember and the next one at the usual time, and *use barrier contraception for the next seven days*. You may need to skip the placebo pills or pill-free days and start on the next active pill. Your doctor/pharmacist can advise. This also applies if you suffer vomiting/diarrhoea while taking the pill, or take medication that inactivates the pill. Always tell your doctor and other healthcare professionals if you are taking hormonal contraception. Stop taking the pill and call a doctor if you suffer severe breathlessness, (or cough up blood), prolonged headaches, severe pain in the chest, stomach or leg, disturbed vision or hearing, or general skin itching or irritation.

ABOVE LEFT

An IUCD can give postsex protection if fitted up to five days (and sometimes even longer) following unprotected sex.

SAFER SEX

BELOW
Discuss condoms with a new partner before you need to use one, to avoid embarrassment later.

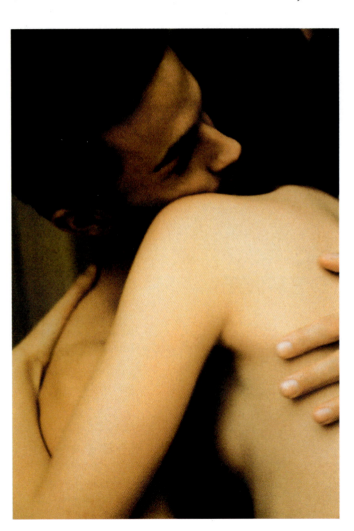

The message is simple, but many people still ignore it. So here it is again, bluntly: HIV/AIDs is fatal. There is no cure. Until a cure is found, the best doctors can do for sufferers is to prescribe drugs to prolong life. A better approach: Don't get it in the first place! You are most likely to catch HIV (the virus that causes AIDs) by:

- Having sex without using a condom.
- Sharing drug needles.

If you don't want to catch HIV:
- Use a condom during sex.
- Don't share drug needles.

Always use a condom in the early stages of a mutually exclusive sexual relationship. Use one every time you have sex if you, or a partner, have other sex partners. If you are in a monogamous relationship – and you trust your partner – there may be a time when you decide to dispense with protection. No one can tell you how soon this should be. You must trust your intuition. If you have any doubts, continue using condoms. If your partner objects, explain your reasons. If your partner still objects, get another partner!

The riskiest sex activities by far are vaginal and anal penetration (without a condom). There may be some risk from oral sex, but it is impossible to say how great. Again, this risk is reduced with a condom (that's why there are flavoured ones). Low-risk sex activities include petting, mutual masturbation and using sex toys such as a vibrator (but don't share).

STRANGER DANGER

It is a fact that must be faced: dangerous men exist, and sooner or later you may meet one. Not every man is a violent sexual predator, but those who *are* often look harmless. Your intuition can help, but it is not foolproof. So make safety your main consideration and limit the risk.

When planning a night out with friends, agree in advance to look out for each other. If you intend drinking, make sure at least one of you stays sober to take care of the rest. It is easy to spike someone's glass with a hypnotic drug or strong liquor so guard each other's drinks. If you think a drink may have been left unattended, no matter how briefly, don't touch it. Don't accept a drink from a stranger unless you see it being mixed at the bar and the barman hands it over to you direct. If you meet someone you'd like to know better, take his number or agree a date but don't leave with him, no matter how great he seems. At the end of the evening, ensure all your friends are present, exit together and share a cab home with those who live near you.

Before you agree to a first date, learn what you can about the person you are meeting. At the very least, check out where he lives and works. This shows he's not bogus but it won't prove he's safe, so you must be on your guard. Arrange to meet in public at a cafe, bar or restaurant, say, not his home. Make sure others know where you are. If you are not within a short walk of home, have your mobile and the number of a reputable taxi firm with you – plus the fare. Avoid drugs and limit your drinking; excess alcohol leads to risky behaviour you may regret. Never leave your drink unattended. If you need to go to the bathroom, finish your drink first, or ask for a fresh one when you return. If a drink is waiting when you get back, don't touch it. If you feel uneasy about a situation – even if you can't say exactly why – just leave.

After a few dates, if you decide to have sex, make sure you have condoms with you and insist on using them for penetrative intercourse. Don't be coerced into anything you do not like, or are not ready for. In particular, don't agree to bondage or other sexual practices that leave you vulnerable until you know you can trust the person.

SEXUALLY TRANSMITTED DISEASES

There are many different sexually transmitted infections (STIs). Some, like HIV and syphilis, can be fatal. Not all cause symptoms but all put health and fertility at risk. If there is a risk you may be infected, visit a genito-urinary medicine (GUM) clinic. Treatment is confidential and you can remain anonymous. If you are diagnosed with an STI you should inform your sexual partner and he or she should visit the clinic too. Possible symptoms include:

- Abnormal discharge or odour from the penis or vagina.
- Pain, soreness, redness or itching around the genital/anal area.
- Pain during sex or when urinating.
- Lower abdominal pain.
- Painful sores/abnormal growths around the mouth, genitals or anus.

FEMALE SEXUAL PROBLEMS

Soreness or mild pain during sex is a common problem for women, due to overenthusiastic lovemaking or lack of vaginal lubrication and/or thinning of the vaginal tissues, especially in later life. Liberal use of a suitable lubricating gel can help. More severe pain may be due to inflammatory conditions such as cystitis (affecting the bladder), bartholinitis (affecting the Bartholin's glands, on either side of the vaginal entrance), an STI (see pages 120–1) or a gynaecological condition such as endometriosis. Pain that is persistent or severe should always be referred to a doctor. Ignored, it could lead to infertility and may be life-threatening. Treatment depends on the underlying disorder.

A condition called vaginismus causes the vaginal walls to spasm painfully whenever a penis, finger or vibrator is inserted. The problem may be due to anxiety, guilt or past trauma that has caused a woman to link sex with pain. The following self-help technique can be effective. The woman spends time on her own learning to relax her vaginal muscles while she explores her body by touch.

BELOW RIGHT
With a caring partner who shows patience and tenderness, most women can reach the level of arousal needed to climax.

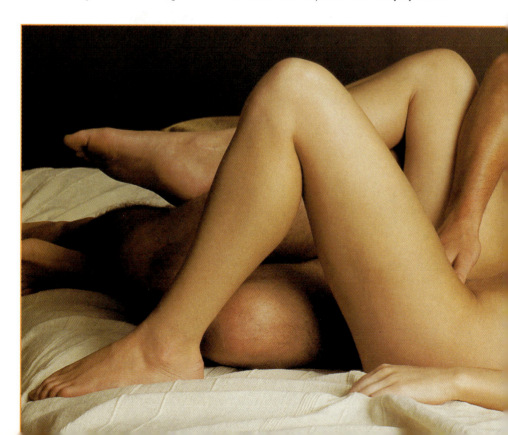

FEMALE SEXUAL PROBLEMS

Her partner is then encouraged to join her, caressing her body gently, helping her to build up trust, but without progressing to intercourse until she no longer tenses at his touch. A doctor or therapist may provide special plastic rods (vaginal trainers) varying from finger-width to vibrator-size. The woman learns to relax enough to insert the narrowest, slowly progressing to the widest. When ready for intercourse, she should adopt positions such as woman on top and side by side that allow her more control over the pace and depth of penetration.

Women may sometimes lose interest in sex (sexual desire disorder), find it difficult to get sexually excited (sexual arousal disorder) or become aroused but fail to achieve satisfaction (orgasmic disorder). The solution may be to spend more time establishing a romantic mood or environment, and on kissing and foreplay and experimenting with different forms of stimulation, including massage and various sexual positions.

Sometimes female problems are signs of deep-seated relationship issues that need to be talked through, perhaps with the aid of a relationship counsellor. Techniques such as sensate focus (see page 125) can help to re-establish an emotional bond between partners. Other causes include stress, anxiety, or the side effect of a physical disorder or drugs (medicinal and recreational). Medication may help in some cases, but attempts to produce a female version of *sildenafil* ('Viagra'), which has been effective for some male sexual problems, have proved unsuccessful.

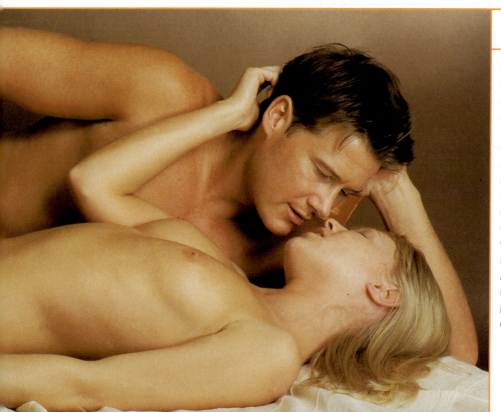

BRIDGE TECHNIQUE

If a woman finds it difficult to reach orgasm through penetrative sex, therapists recommend trying the 'bridge technique'. Here, the man stimulates his partner using hands, mouth and/or vibrator until she is close to orgasm. He then enters her and brings her to orgasm by penile thrusting, with additional manual stimulation if necessary. As with all problems of a sexual nature, this requires patience and understanding on both sides.

MALE SEXUAL PROBLEMS

BELOW
Male sexual problems can often be resolved with the help of a loving and understanding partner.

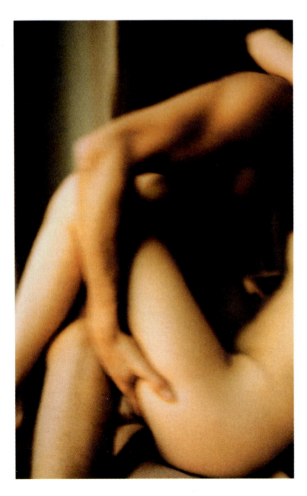

The two most common male sexual problems are premature ejaculation and impotence (erectile dysfunction). Premature ejaculation sometimes has an underlying psychological cause. If so, your doctor or a sex therapist may be able to help. Many of the techniques and positions described in this book, including the squeeze technique (see page 19), can help delay orgasm in men. Having ejaculated once, through foreplay, oral sex or intercourse, a man may find he can delay his orgasm during subsequent sexual activity long enough to satisfy his partner.

Impotence, the inability to achieve or maintain an erection, can have physical and emotional causes. If a man can never achieve an erection, even during sleep or when he wakes up in the morning, the problem may be a physical one, for example due to a disorder such as diabetes or a side effect of medications or recreational drugs, including cigarettes and alcohol. If you suspect this is the cause, a doctor should be consulted.

If the problem only occurs during sexual intercourse, there may be an underlying emotional or psychological cause. Stress, overwork, financial worries and relationship problems all impact on the 'sexual mind'. Often a feeling of being under pressure to perform can cause anxiety-related impotence. If a man fails to achieve an erection once, he may feel under greater pressure the next time, leading to a downward spiral. Medications, such as *sildenafil* ('Viagra'), or vacuum pump devices can be effective. Taking a more relaxed attitude to sex, spending time simply kissing, touching, stroking and cuddling, without necessarily having sex, can help overcome performance anxiety. This is the principle behind the sensate focus technique (see opposite). If you're in a loving relationship, with patience, understanding, some knowledge and perhaps expert help, you can usually work through these problems together.

MALE SEXUAL PROBLEMS | 125

SENSATE FOCUS

This technique is prescribed by sex therapists. It avoids performance pressure and helps enhance the emotional bond. But couples also need to look at the relationship as a whole, talking through areas of conflict and spending more time together. Sensate focus involves twice-weekly sessions, initially of 20 minutes and slowly building up to an hour. It is carried out in three or more stages, but without deadlines. Couples continue with each stage for as long as necessary. Depending on the couple's progress, the therapist suggests when it might be appropriate to move on to the next stage.

- *Stage one* Here, the couple take turns to touch and stroke each other, avoiding sexual areas such as breasts and genitals, simply enjoying touching and being touched, without engaging in sex. After a few weeks they will be encouraged to seek out new tactile sensations, for example through massage, and by using different materials.

- *Stage two* Continuing as before, the couple progress to simultaneous touching. Over the weeks they can include sexual areas, such as the breasts, and later the genitals, but stop short of arousal. They then progress to mutual masturbation leading to orgasm.

- *Stage three* The couple continue as before, progressing to penetration when ready, but without movement and not leading to orgasm. Over the weeks to come, they can include thrusting movements, finally leading to orgasm, but only if and when they choose. By the end of treatment, the couple should have a more loving and sharing attitude to sex – and the relationship – without feeling under pressure to climax.

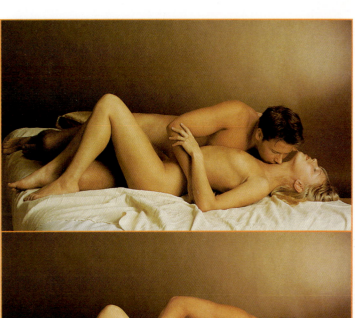
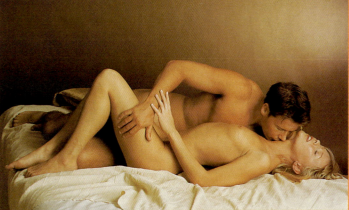
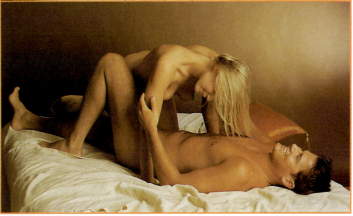

INDEX

A
adventurous sex 93–4
alcohol 38
anus 14, 15
aphrodisiacs 37–8
arousal 20
atmosphere 36

B
barrier methods 116–7
biting 105, 106
bondage 102–3
'bow' sexual position 94–5
breasts 13, 16, 57
bridge technique 123
Burton, Sir Richard 10
butt plugs 110
buttocks 15

C
cap 117
caressing 84
cleanliness 24–5
clitoris 13, 16, 67
clothing 41, 99
condoms 116, 117, 120
contraception 116–19
cunnilingus 65–9

D
dating 36, 121
delaying ejaculation 19
diaphragm 117
divine sex 111–2

E
ejaculation 19
embracing 43
erogenous zones
  female 13, 42
  male 15, 42
excitement phase 16
exercise 22–3, 69

F
fantasies 99
feathers 28
feet 57
fellatio 70–3
female
  arousal 20
  bondage 102–3
  cleanliness 25
  cunnilingus 65–9
  domination 102–3
  erogenous zones 13, 42, 56–7
  excitement phase 16
  foreplay 56–7, 59
  masturbation 62
  'missionary position' 78–81
  orgasm 13, 16, 19
  plateau phase 16, 19
  rear-entry position 86–7
  refractory phase 19
  seated position 88–91
  sex organs 12–13
  sexual attraction 34–5
  sexual problems 122–3
  sexual response 21, 41
  side-by-side position 84–5
  skin 13, 28
  standing sex position 91–2
  woman-on-top position 82–3
foreplay 41–2, 56–9

G
G-spot 18

H
HIV/AIDS 120
hormonal contraception 118

I
impotence 124
inner labia 12
inner-thigh stretch 23
intra-uterine contraceptive device (IUCD) 119

K
Kama Sutra 6–9, 24, 27, 32, 33, 37, 38, 51, 53, 56, 64, 73, 74, 77, 86, 92, 97–8, 99, 104, 105
kissing 53–5
knees-to-chest exercise 23

L
lubrication 78

M
male
  arousal 20
  bondage 102–3
  cleanliness 25
  domination 102–3
  ejaculation 19, 124
  erogenous zones 15, 42, 57
  excitement phase 16
  fellatio 70–3
  foreplay 56–7
  impotence 124

masturbation 60, 63
'missionary position' 78–81
orgasm 16, 19
plateau phase 16
premature ejaculation 124
rear-entry position 86–7
refractory phase 19
seated position 88–91
sex organs 14
sexual attraction 34–5
sexual problems 124
sexual response 21
side-by-side position 84–5
standing sex position 91–2
woman-on-top position 82–3
massage 46–9
menstrual cycle 24, 25
'missionary position' 11, 78–81
mutual masturbation 60–3

N
nipple clamps 110

O
oils 47–8, 49
oral sex 64–78
orgasm
   female 13, 19
   male 16, 19
outer labia 12, 62

P
partner-aided hip stretch 23
pelvic circles 23
pelvic floor 24
penis 14, 16, 25, 63, 95
perineum 12, 13

pill, the 118, 119
plateau phase 16, 19
pleasure beads 110
positions
   'bow' 94–5
   'missionary position' 11, 78–81
   rear-entry 86–7
   seated 88–91
   side-by-side 84–5
   'spinning top' 95
   standing 91–2
   'turning' 95
   woman-on-top 82–3
premature ejaculation 124
prostrate gland 14

R
rear-entry position 86–7
refractory phase 19
romantic atmosphere 36

S
scratching 105–6
scrotum 14, 16
seated position 88–91
seduction 41–2
self-confidence 32
sensate focus 125
sex games 100
sex organs
   female 12–13
   male 14
sex toys 108–10
sexual attraction 32–5
sexual environment 38, 40
sexual problems
   female 122–3
sexual response 21

sexually transmitted diseases 121
Shakti 9
Shiva 9
side-by-side position 84–5
'sixty-nine' position 74–5
skin 13, 15, 28
smacking 104–5
smell 21, 25, 27, 99
sounds 27
'spinning top' sexual position 95
sponge 117
squats 23
standing sex position 91–2
stroking 28, 79

T
Tantra 9, 111–13
testicles 14
touch 28, 42–3
'turning' sexual position 95
undressing 44–5

V
vagina 13, 16, 25, 62
vaginismus 122–3
Vatsyayana 6, 9, 10, 11, 22, 24, 27,
   34, 38, 53, 54, 77, 86, 95, 104,
   105, 106
vibrators 63, 103, 109
vulva 12–13, 25, 67

W
water 100
woman-on-top position 82–3

ACKNOWLEDGEMENTS

The author would like to express his thanks to photographer Laura Knox, photographic assistant Laura Forrester and make-up artist Sophia Atcha, for their skill, wit and welcome hospitality; models Abigail Toyne, Katie Lawrie, Janie Dickens, Ricky Dearman, Simon Dowling and John Viales for their imagination and boundless enthusiasm; Katrina Dallamore and Bobby Birchall at DW design for their eye-catching layouts; copy editor Jane Donovan for her invaluable insights and suggestions, and last but definitely not least, executive editor Lisa Dyer, for her patience, support and much-needed encouragement.

PICTURE CREDITS

The publishers would like to thank the following sources for their kind permission to reproduce the pictures in this book.

AKG London: 101,115; /Jean-Louis Nou: 4, 9, 26, 97, 106

The Bridgeman Art Library: Archives Charmet: 19, 31, 37, 82, 87; /Dinodia Picture Agency: 6, 7; /Fitzwilliam Museum, University of Cambridge: 93, 117; / Private Collection: 51, 55, 58, 77, 78; /Raiput School: 14

Carlton Books Ltd: Laura Knox: 2-3, 8, 11, 22, 23, 29, 30, 33, 35, 39, 42, 50, 60, 66, 67, 68-69, 70, 71, 72-73, 74, 75, 76, 80, 81, 83, 85, 86, 92, 93, 94, 95, 96, 104, 105, 107, 112, 113, 114, 119, 122-23; 125; /Peter Pugh-Cook: 18, 53, 62, 63, 90, 98, 99, 102, 108, 109, 110; /Alan Randall: 46, 47

Photolibrary.com: Photo Alto: 5, 10, 12, 13, 15, 17, 20, 21, 25, 27, 40, 43, 44, 45, 48, 49, 52, 54, 56, 57, 59, 79, 87, 88, 89, 103, 111, 118, 120, 124

Werner Forman Archive: Private Collection: 64

Every effort has been made to acknowledge correctly and contact the source and/or copyright holder of each picture and Carlton Books Limited apologizes for any unintentional errors or omissions that will be corrected in future editions of this book.